Continuing Care of Sick Children:
Examining the impact of chronic illness

Continuing Care of Sick Children: Examining the impact of chronic illness

by

Christine Cooper

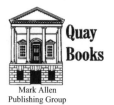

Quay Books

Mark Allen
Publishing Group

Quay Books, a division of Mark Allen Publishing Ltd,
Jesses Farm, Snow Hill, Dinton, Salisbury, Wiltshire SP3 5HN

British Library Cataloguing-in-Publication Data
A catalogue record for this book is available from the British Library

ISBN 1 85642 032 9
© Mark Allen Publishing Limited 1999

Printed in the United Kingdom by The Cromwell Press, Trowbridge,
Wiltshire

Contents

v

Contributors

Christine Cooper, MSc, BSc (Hons), RGN, RSCN, NT, is Principal Lecturer (Paediatric) at the University of Central England in Birmingham. She has a wide experience of caring for children with chronic illness and currently co-ordinates and teaches the continuing care of children with chronic illnesses on a wide variety of modules at diploma, degree, and masters level.

Alison Twycross, RGN, RMN, RSCN, MSc, DMS Cert Ed, Lecturer in Nursing Studies at Nottingham University, has contributed *Chapter 4*. She has researched and written a number of papers on the subject of pain in children. In addition, she has recently published a book examining pain in children from a multi-disciplinary perspective and is currently undertaking a PhD, examining nurses' attitudes to children in pain.

Linda Kilshaw, BA, MA, RGN, RSCN, NDN, Reg CT, RNT, Senior Lecturer (Child Health/Ethics) at John Moores University, Liverpool, is co-author of *Chapter 7*. She has extensive experience in children's nursing and teaches a wide variety of children's pre- and post-registration courses. She is currently undertaking a PhD for which she is examining negotiation and partnership with families with a chronically ill child.

Preface

The body of knowledge on the effects of chronic disorders on the child and family has been growing, particularly over the last 25 years. However, much of the focus has been to provide treatment and management of specific chronic disorders. Although this approach mirrors the way medical paediatric specialities are organised with research focused on the differences between the disease processes, there has been increasing recognition that this approach has obscured the common stresses and consequences of chronic illness for the child and family (Eiser, 1993; Bradford, 1997). Thus this book aims to explore chronic illness from a perspective that identifies the common reactions and problems that may arise for children and families and the relevance this has for practitioners within the field of child health.

The focus on chronic disease has largely been the result of medical and technological advances in the western world. Over the last fifty years there has been a dramatic reduction in the mortality rate in children, particularly as a result of improved treatments of infectious diseases, technological advances and the improvement in public and private preventative health care strategies. Mortality rates estimates indicate a fall from 870 per 100, 000 of all children between 1 and 14 years in 1900 to 33 per 100,000 in 1987 (Newacheck and Taylor, 1992). While the overall incidence of chronic illnesses has not changed to the same degree, there has been an increase in the prevalence, and the categories of chronic illness conditions are rapidly expanding. However, statistics for chronic illness are at best estimates largely due to the confusion of what constitutes a chronic illness. Thus, some of the issues of incidence and prevalence will be explored in *Chapter 1* to provide an introduction to key issues and a framework for further exploration of the impact of chronic illness on the child and family.

Estimates of survival rates have shown a considerable change as children with chronic illnesses, who once died in infancy, are now surviving to adulthood and have to cope with often continual and increasingly complex treatment regimens. The impact this has on a child's development varies according to the age, effects of the disease and treatment, and family characteristics. There has always been an acknowledgement that care should provide a good quality of life, however, this tended to be through management of the ongoing symptoms, and acute episodes of the disorder and the developmental needs were secondary. While treatment management still continues to ensure that children achieve a 'good' quality of life, there is a greater appreciation of the need to help children achieve their developmental potential. The emphasis is on managing the care by balancing the effect of the disease and the potential benefits of treatment against the ongoing growth and development needs. There is a need to evaluate the impact of chronic illness on the development of a child with such an illness in order to enable them to reach their potential. This is explored in *Chapters 2* and *3*.

The diagnosis and treatment of a chronic illness can lead to a number of adverse consequences for the child, including pain. Although not all chronic disorders result in chronic pain, this is the experience of some children and many children with chronic illness can face a battery of tests and procedures to confirm diagnosis and sometimes complex and painful treatments. The impact of chronic and acute episodes of pain for the child and family with a chronic illness is explored in *Chapter 4*.

The implications of a diagnosis of a chronic illness has far-reaching consequences for the family. Chronic illness produces both emotional and practical consequences but the impact varies depending on the severity of the condition, the effects of treatment, and the family dynamics which influence the ability of each family to 'cope'. Although we need to guard against assumptions that negative consequences are an inevitable feature of chronic illness, the added burden of care as a result of the chronically ill child may lead to tension within the family. Stress may be created that affects the family's ability to adapt to the resulting changes to family life. Some of the factors that influence parental coping are explored in *Chapter 5*.

Theoretical models that have attempted to predict the adaptation or maladaptation of the family to chronic illness have been limited due to the complex interaction of factors which affect family coping. Although the models are useful in identifying some of the issues for families it is difficult to predict the consequences for the child and family. However, the models available do provide a way of visualising the complexity and interconnecting issues which influence the adaptation of children and families. There are a number of models in common use to explain the adaptation of families to chronic illness. *Chapter 6* aims to provide an overview of some of the theoretical models as a backdrop to an evaluation of the complex interaction of factors that have an impact on the child's and the family's adaptation to chronic illness.

The consequences of chronic illness for the child and family mean a revolution in the ways in which they cope with the everyday challenges of care. The family bears the burden of care, so if nurses are to support the family it must be through partnership and negotiation which is explored in *Chapter 7*.

The impact of chronic illness on the child and family is complex and this book can not possibly explore all permutations. However, it is hoped the book will help practitioners, involved in the care of children, to appreciate the impact that chronic illness can have on the child and family.

References

Bradford R (1997) *Children, families and chronic disease. Psychological models and methods of care.* Routledge, London

Eiser C (1993) *Growing up with a chronic disease. The impact on children and their families.* Jessica Kingsley Publishers, London

Newacheck PW, Taylor WR (1992) Childhood chronic illness: prevalence, severity and impact. *Am J Public Health* **82**(3): 364–71

1
Overview of chronic illness: issues relevant to chronic illness in children

Introduction

> *'It's always with you, you can't put it aside and think it'll be better tomorrow because you know every day you have to go through the same routines all over again, feeling terrible, drugs, physio... it never goes away... .'*

(Paul, aged 20 years, cystic fibrosis)

This quote gives some indication of what it must be like to have a chronic illness. Yet the term 'chronic' incorporates a wide variety of disorders which differ in their specific limitations and impact on the child and family. However, they share a common theme which is captured in how Paul talks of his illness; 'they can not be cured' (Eiser, 1993). Although there have been a number of medical advances in treatment that aim to control the effects of the disease and promote an improved quality of life for the child, they do not generally offer a cure.

Children with chronic illness do not represent a homogeneous group in that there is infinite diversity amongst them in terms of:

- the nature of the disorder
- progression and severity of the disease
- cultural attitudes and beliefs
- social circumstamces
- ability of child and family to adapt
- aspirations of child and family.

However, they all share the need to have the technical and medical aspects of their care balanced with their need, and that of their families, for some sort of 'normal life'.

Impact of diagnosis

> *'You will never forget the words. For as long as you live,*

*through the sad times and the happy times, the words will
always come back to you. Those first words the doctor spoke
to you, telling you there was a problem with your child. The
way you accept and the way you begin to deal with the
situation starts with the first words you hear.'*

(Swirydczuk, 1991, p.34)

The hurt behind these words shows us how the diagnosis of a chronic
illness brings with it an 'irreversible change in the life of the child and
family' (Davis, 1993) as they learn to cope with the impact of the
disorder and its treatment.

As Eiser (1990) comments:

*'The diagnosis of chronic disease in children sets the stage
for a revolution in the way of life, experienced by patient and
family. Implications are far reaching, affecting everyday
routines, hopes and ambitions and the relationships both
between family members and with the outside world.'* (p.1)

Significance of the problem

The number of children and families coping with disabilities is set to
rise as advances in healthcare improve the lives of children with chronic
illnesses. Thus, there is an increasing number of children who once
would have died from their disability, now surviving into adulthood
(Newacheck and Taylor, 1992).

Despite the rising numbers, children with chronic illnesses are still
a relatively neglected group within society. This is partly due to the
small number of children with specific chronic illnesses and the rarity
of some conditions when compared to the numbers of chronically ill
adults (Perrin and Maclean, 1988). However, figures such as 10 to 15
per cent of children (1 per cent of the total population under 18 years)
are frequently cited (Gortmaker, 1985; Wiesland *et al*, 1992,
Thompson and Gustafason, 1996) and it is estimated that 10 per cent of
these children have problems that interfere with their ability to carry out
tasks appropriate to their chronological age (Pless and Perrin, 1985;
Thompson and Gustafason, 1996). This ten per cent could account for a
million children with severe problems that affect their daily lives

(Perrin and Maclean, 1988), which is a significant number of children who will need treatment and support to cope with the impact of a chronic illness.

Incidence/prevalence of chronic illness

Despite the number of children with chronic illness the knowledge of the incidence, prevalence and demographic distribution is limited (Starfield, 1991).

Accurate statistics which indicate incidence and prevalence are not widely available for all chronic conditions.

Incidence is defined as the number of new occurrences of disease per unit of population during a specified period.

Prevalence is defined as the number of new and continuing cases.

Some chronic illnesses of special interest, such as asthma and cancers, are more thoroughly documented and have more complete data, but this is not true for rarer conditions such as sickle-cell disease and haemophilia. The problem arises out of the limited number of research studies available, the varied choice of sample populations and the inconsistency of classification of some disorders (such as epilepsy), resulting in widely differing estimates of incidence and prevalence for specific chronic illnesses. Thus, statistics are usually estimates of the scope of the problem drawing on international data, which means that demographic trends in chronic diseases in children are difficult to predict.

Table 1.1 (on *page 4*) identifies not only the wide variety of disorders but also the age of onset, incidence and survival rate of the children with those chronic disorders.

Incidence of chronic illness

While there have been some changes in the incidence of some conditions such as asthma (Strachan *et al*, 1993), diabetes (Burden *et al*, 1989; Gardner *et al*, 1997), and inflammatory bowel disease (Montgomery *et al*, 1997), the information available indicates that there is little evidence for a significant change in the overall incidence

Table 1.1: The incidence and estimated survival rate (to 20 years of age) of children with chronic illnesses

Chronic disease	Age of onset	Estimated incidence per 1000 live births	Estimated % survival rates to 20 years
Arthritis (JCA) (Simmons *et al*, 1996)	Variable. Peak onset 2–5 yrs, 9 yrs and 12 yrs	0.1	Normal
Asthma (Strachan *et al*, 1993	Variable normally 1–2 yrs	13.1 (definitive diagnosis)	Similar to normal
Chronic renal disease	1–15 yrs	2.0	Few fatalities
Cancer (all sites) (Bleyer, 1990)	Variable	14.0	60–65% for 5 yrs post diagnosis
Cystic fibrosis (Fitzsimmons, 1994)	Birth. Diagnosis may not be made until later. 80% of children diagnosed by 4 yrs	0.5	70%
Diabetes mellitus (Burden *et al*, 1989; Gardner *et al*, 1997)	0–15 yrs. Peak 10–12 yrs for girls. Peak 12–14 yrs for boys	1.9	95%
Epilepsy and seizures (Berg *et al*, 1996)	1–5 yrs febrile convulsions. Epilepsy seizures are rare under 8 yrs	Under 10 yrs 1.7 over 10 yrs 3.3	Normal
Eczema and skin allergies (Newacheck and Taylor, 1992)	Variable	32.9	Normal
Heart disease (congenital)	88% by first yr	8.0	52% to 15 yrs
Inflammatory bowel disorders Ulcerative colitis Crohn's disease (Montgomery *et al*, 1997)	Early adolescence. Rare under 9 yrs	6.0	Normal
Haemophilia (Goldsmith, 1994)	90% by 3–4 yrs	0.13 (males)	Relatively normal
Leukaemia (Swartz *et al*, 1994)	Variable	0.032	40–70% survival rate (depending on diagnosis)
Sickle-cell disease	End of first yr	0.4	Normal

Updated and adapted from Gortmaker (1985). The data for the table is extracted from a variety of sources and is a best estimate from currently available data in order to give a complete picture. Please note that the data is based on estimates from small population studies and from other countries such as the United States.

of chronic illnesses (Thompson and Gustavson, 1996). However, the prevalence of chronic illness doubled from one per cent to two per cent between the 1960s and the 1980s (Gortmaker and Sappenfield, 1984). Although the overall prevalence for chronic illness appears to be increasing, it is difficult to provide accurate figures to support this as there is no central database on chronic illness in children. The government publication, *The Health of Our Children* (Bootling, 1996), bears testimony to this as the estimates of childhood morbidity in it have been inferred from statistics on specific disorders. However, the increase in prevalence of chronic disorders means that children who would previously have died from their illnesses are now surviving with increasingly complex and disabling problems (Newacheck and Taylor, 1992).

Prevalence of chronic illness

The evidence available indicates that the patterns of prevalence for chronic illness in children is not uniform for all chronic disorders. Although there has been little change in the survival rate for disorders such as epilepsy or renal disease, other disorders have seen remarkable improvements. Children with cystic fibrosis have had a sevenfold increase in survival to 21 years and there has been a twofold or more increase for leukaemia and other cancers (Thompson and Gustavson, 1996). Several factors have influenced the change in prevalence. They include:

- improved early diagnosis and treatment which has increased life expectancy
- improved survival of low birth weight and premature infants with complex problems
- the survival of children with new diagnosed conditions (ie. cancers, HIV positive/AIDS)
- changes in environmental factors such as pollution (an example of this is the increasing number of children being diagnosed with asthma)
- changes in ethnic and social background. Poverty, particularly, can affect the resources and management of the disorder and has been directly linked to the prevalence of a disorder.

However, there is some confusion regarding what can be classified as a chronic illness.

Defining chronic illness

In examining the literature there are a number of definitions of chronic illness which are often quoted, but the most widely accepted is Mattson's (1972), who suggested:

> *'Chronic illness refers to a disorder with a protracted course which can be progressive and fatal or associated with a relatively normal life span despite impaired physical and medical functioning. Such a disease frequently shows periods of acute exacerbation requiring intensive medical attention.'* (p.5)

What is considered to be a chronic disorder has been extended as a result of the increased prevalence of chronic disabling conditions, and the definition of 'chronic' can include developmental problems such as mental retardation, blindness and deafness. There has been some debate about whether mental retardation or congenital disability can be incorporated into discussions about the impact of chronic illness on children and their families. Some surveys incorporate both chronic illness and congenital disabilities as one group (Boyle *et al*, 1994), while other surveys evaluate chronic illness as a single category, considering chronic illness as distinct from developmental disabilities (Thomson and Gustatafson, 1996). In part this is due to the difficulties of comparing the problems of children who have chronic illness with those who have congenital disabilities. A child with a chronic illness may have a disability, but a child with a disability is not by definition ill. However, there is some overlap when considering the impact of a chronic illness, disability or handicap on the child and the family.

Disability, disease and handicap

Often the terms 'disease', 'disability' and 'handicap' are used interchangeably when discussing chronic illness. 'Disease' or 'illness' generally refers to the biological basis of the disorder, and 'disability' and 'handicap' to the behavioural consequences.

To distinguish between 'disability' and 'handicap', the World Health Organisation (1980) defines 'disability' as 'the consequence of impairment', and 'handicap' as 'the social disadvantage of disability'.

For example, a chronic illness such as AIDS may prevent a child from being able to fulfil either growth and development potential or normal social roles as a result of an increasing disability, but it is society's attitudes which determine the impact or degree of the handicap.

Chronic illness

A chronic illness resulting from biological processes can lead to increasing disability or handicap for a child. Although medicine may provide treatment to control the symptoms, it does not generally offer a cure.

Pless and Pinkerton (1975) suggested that an illness could be considered chronic when it persisted for longer than three months in one year, or required a period of continuous hospitalisation for more than one month. Although this definition is broad and can include trauma injuries which require extended hospitalisation, it does highlight that chronic illness affects the life of a child over a period of time. While three months may not appear to be a long time, and children may be fairly resilient in overcoming the effects of hospitalisation or protracted illness, the consequences may still have a significant impact on a child's development, particularly if the problems occur during critical developmental periods in the child's life.

The effects of a chronic illness can vary considerably for, although chronic illness may be characterised as a group of disorders, the features of the disorders can vary enormously.

Characteristics of chronic illness

Eiser (1990) suggested that some of the differences between chronic illnesses can include:
- the cause (aetiology) of the disease
- the manifestations of the disorder, that is, the signs and symptoms
- the stability and predictability of the disease process, in turn affecting the ability to anticipate periods of acute exacerbation of the disorder
- the treatment regimes
- the threat to life
- the demands imposed by the treatments which affect daily routines.

The varying characteristics have created some debate regarding how to categorise the disorders. In examining the literature a number of approaches to categorising chronic illness are evident.

Categorical and non-categorical approaches

Categorical approach

The **categorical** approach suggests that all chronic disorders vary so much in terms of symptoms, diagnosis and treatment that each disease must be considered unique. This approach has largely been adopted by medical research and has been useful as it has allowed the advances in diagnosis and treatment of such disorders as diabetes and cystic fibrosis which have significantly improved the lives of many children. However, the specialism has resulted in a fragmented approach to care (Perrin, 1994), and it was not clear from the available research how far the problems identified in each category, for example diabetes or asthma, were the result of the specific disease or a problem due to the chronic nature of the disorder.

Non-categorical approach

Advocates of a **non-categorical** approach suggest that exploring individual diseases fails to appreciate the similarities of the experiences of many families (Stein and Jessop, 1982), such as family disruption as a result of care and the impact of treatments on family resources. For example, a child who is in hospital faces days lost from school whether or not the reason was due to an asthma attack or a sickle-cell crisis. A non-categorical approach looks at the common experiences of children with chronic illnesses and their families, and the impact these may have on the families and the children's growth and development. This approach has the benefit of promoting positive policies for children with rare conditions, as it is easier to recommend the provision of educational support and to justify the expenditure for children with chronic illness than to focus on an individual condition which affects very few children (Eiser, 1993).

Modified approach

It is very difficult to take an 'either/or' position (Thompson and Gustafson, 1996), as both categorical and non-categorical approaches have value in developing strategies to improve the quality of life for the child and family. Pless and Perrin (1985) suggest a **modified** approach which aims to identify both the illness' specific characteristics and the generic processes of adaptation to chronic illnesses. This provides a way to consider the general adaptation processes of children with chronic illnesses while utilising specific examples of how these may differ with specific disorders. In this way it is hoped to develop a framework which explores the factors that affect a child's ability to cope with chronic illness generally, but also develops strategies for specific conditions. This two-pronged (modified) approach may enable practitioners and researchers to develop a broader strategy to improve the quality of life for the child and family.

The effects of chronic illness

This book utilises a modified approach in examining the impact of chronic illness on the child and family. The aim is to explore some of the common factors that influence the development of the child and the adaptation of the family to chronic illness while acknowledging that the impact is modified by the condition and the characteristics of the child and family.

Stress for the child and family

Chronic illness is a recognised source of stress in the life of the child and family (Perrin and Maclean, 1988). Research has tended to emphasise the potential causes of developmental delay or 'maladjustment' as a result of the interference with normal development (Perrin and Gerrity, 1984). Care must be taken in interpreting the literature, as empirical evidence is limited and it is often difficult to determine whether the cause of the delay is as a result of the chronic illness. It is estimated children with chronic illness are 1.5 to 3 times more likely to show problems of developmental delay when compared to their healthy peers (Pless, 1984). The reasons for the delay are not always clear, but an illness can place restrictions on the child and family. Thomas (1987) suggested chronic illness:

> *'... interferes with the individual's ability to function fully in the environment...'* (p.5)

A chronically ill child faces consequences of a disorder which their 'healthy' peers do not. Jessop and Stein (1988) outlined a number of potential problems including:

- a change in their diet to control symptoms
- dependence on medication
- dependence on technology, such as intravenous drugs or enteral feeds
- ongoing treatment at home.

Such problems can occupy a lot of time and energy both for the child undergoing the treatment and the family which bears the burden of care. The additional demands of treatment and care create stress which is superimposed on the 'normal' demands of parenting and childhood.

The impact on the child and family

It is difficult to predict the impact of a chronic illness on a child and family as chronic illness incorporates such a wide variety of disorders (see *Table 1.1*) and the severity of the problems of disorders can vary enormously. For example, asthma for one child can mean having to cope with occasional bouts of wheeziness, while for another it may mean 'brittle asthma' which could necessitate frequent hospitalisation.

Such problems can influence a child's interaction with the environment and have been seen as a potential source of stress and so a factor increasing the likelihood of developmental delay. Chronic illness adds another dimension to a child's experience, but the impact of the diagnosis varies according to the consequences and meaning of the chronic condition and the ability of the child and family to 'cope'.

Coping with chronic illness

Coping is seen as positive and 'adaptive' (Rose and Thomas, 1987) when both the child and the family are able to deal actively with the problems either by changing themselves in order to 'fit in', or by changing the physical, social or emotional environment around them.

Coping may be defined as: the ability to modify and utilise a variety of strategies to deal positively with everyday challenges.

Logically it would follow that the more difficult the situation, as a result of the severity of a chronic illness, the more difficult it would be to 'cope'. However, as Perrin (1994) has noted, there is no direct correlation between coping and severity of the disease, as the effect of the disorder on the child and family may be modified by a number of factors. These can include:

- social expectation
- support of friends and family
- age and development of child at diagnosis
- presentation of symptoms
- ability to treat the disorder
- consequences of diagnosis and treatment
- characteristics of the child
- family characteristics.

Pless and Pinkerton (1975) suggested that the impact of the disorder on the child and family is perhaps more significant than the disorder itself. The procedures for diagnosis and subsequent treatment of the disorder can be time-consuming and financially and emotionally draining, and although the treatment may offer relief from symptoms, it does not generally offer a cure. Many of the children will have a relatively 'normal' lifespan, thus the impact of the management of the chronic illness needs to be considered together with the most appropriate strategies to enable the child and family to 'cope' with a potential lifetime of the consequences of a chronic illness.

Focus of care

The impact of a chronic illness on a child and family should not be underestimated. Children with chronic illnesses have unique social and health needs, as chronic illness is not only ongoing but also unpredictable. Children go through periods of acute exacerbation and also remissions, both of which are superimposed on their growth and development needs.

With the increasing prevalence of children with chronic disorders and complex disabling problems there has been a significant shift both in the approach to care and in considering the quality of life of the child and family (Perrin, 1994). It may be argued that quality of life has always been a consideration of care, however more recently there has been an increased awareness of both the impact of chronic illness and its treatment on the families and children's lives, and children's ongoing developmental needs (Bradford, 1997).

Quality of life

Quality of life is an elusive concept and there are a wide variety of definitions and a number of tools to measure what is considered to affect a child's and a family's well-being (Renwick *et al*, 1996). However, quality of life remains subjective and difficult to measure, as each individual copes with and perceives problems according to how they affect their everyday lives and the importance they attach to that interference. For example, for children how 'staying in' as a result of chronic illness is perceived to affect their quality of life depends on whether they like 'staying in', or on whether they have favourite activities inside such as computer games, and the importance they place on going outside with their friends.

Quality of life may be defined as: the areas (domains) of psychological, social and physical factors that interact and affect an individual's perception of their ability to enjoy and cope with the demands of everyday life.

Thus, in exploring chronic illness and quality-of-life issues, it is important to evaluate how the illness affects all 'domains' of an individual's life. It is perhaps more difficult to evaluate quality-of-life issues with children who are still developing and cannot always articulate their thoughts and feelings. However, where possible, this should not prevent the inclusion of the child in decisions about treatment options. Although survival of the child is paramount, some consideration must be given to the child and family so that the benefits are balanced against the negative impact of treatment on the quality of life. For example, the treatment options for a child with cancer may have similar prognoses and the choice generally is one of medical needs or preference, but to ensure an optimum quality of life, the choice must be influenced by the effects of the treatment offered and the ability of family and child to 'cope' with the physical, social or psychological consequences.

Conclusion

It may be argued that the aim of care for children with chronic illnesses has always been to minimise the effect of the disease and so enable the child to enhance their quality of life, but more recently there has been a greater consideration of the effects on the family and the child's development (Eiser, 1993; Bradford, 1997). The current focus of care must incorporate a developmental framework that seeks to enable children to overcome any barriers that may hinder them reaching their potential as they grow into adulthood.

Summary

1   With the prevalence of children with chronic illness on the increase, practitioners are likely to see more families and children with complex and disabling problems.

2   The symptoms, diagnosis and treatment of chronic disorders can vary significantly, but the experiences for families can be similar across disorders.

3   Chronic illness cannot generally be cured and so the emphasis of care needs to evaluate the impact on the quality of life for the child and family.

Implications for practice

1   Practitioners need to be aware that although conditions vary, some of the experiences of parents with chronically ill children may be very similar, such as financial worries, emotional impact of diagnosis, and the day-to-day demands of care. Although there may be few specific conditions within a single region, it may be possible to support families by developing

strategies to cope with physical, financial and emotional stress.

2   The aim of care should be to provide support and care in order to promote as 'normal' a family life as possible. Strategies for care must balance the benefits of treatment against the negative impact on the child and family.

References

Berg AT, Testa FM, Levey SR *et al* (1996) The epidemiology of epilepsy. *Neurol Clin* **14**(2): 383–98

Bleyer WA (1990) The impact of childhood cancer on the United States and the world. *J Cancer Clinics* **40**: 355–67

Bootling B ed. (1996) *The Health of Our Children. Decennial Supplement.* OPCS, HMSO, London

Boyle CA, Decoufle P, Yeargin-Allsopp Y (1994) Prevalence and health impact of developmental disabilities in US children. *Pediatrics* **93**(3): 399–403

Bradford R (1997) *Children, families and chronic disease. Psychological models and methods of care.* Routledge Publications, London

Burden AC, Hearnshaw JR, Swift PGF (1989) Diabetes Mellitus: an increasing incidence. *Diabet Med* **6**: 334–6

Davis H (1993) *Counselling Parents of Children With Chronic Illness and Disability.* British Psychological Society, London

Eiser C (1990) *Chronic Childhood Disease: An introduction to psychological theory and research.* Cambridge University Press, Cambridge

Eiser C (1993) *Growing Up With Chronic Disease. The Impact on Children and Their Families.* Jessica Kingsley Publishers, London

Fitzsimmons SC (1994) The changing epidemiology of cystic fibrosis. *Curr Probl Pediatr* **24**(5): 171–9

Gardner S, Bingley PJ, Sawtell PA *et al* (1997) Rising incidence of insulin dependant diabetes in children under 5 years in the Oxford Region: time trend analysis. *Br Med J* **315**: 713–7

Goldsmith J (1994) *Haemophilia: Current Medical Management.* National Haemophilia Foundation, New York

Gortmaker SL (1985) Demography of chronic childhood diseases. In: Hobbs N, Perrin JM eds. (1985) *Issues in the Care of Children With Chronic Illness.* Jossey Bass, San Francisco

Gortmaker SL, Sappenfield (1984) Chronic childhood disorders: prevalence and impact. *Pediatr Clin North Am* **31**(1): 3–18

Jessop DJ, Stein RK (1988) Essential concepts in the care of children with chronic illness. *Pediatrics* **15**: 5–12

Mattson A (1972) Long term physical illness in childhood: a challenge to psycho-social adaptation. *Pediatrics* **50**: 5

Montgomery SM, Pounder RE, Wakefield AJ (1997) Infant mortality and the incidence of inflamatory bowel disease. *Lancet* **349**: 472–3

Newacheck PW, Taylor WR (1992) Childhood chronic illness; prevalence, severity and impact. *Am J Public Health* **82**(3): 364–71

Perrin JM (1994) Health care reform and the special needs of children. *Pediatrics* **93**(3): 504–6

Perrin EC, Gerrity BS (1984) Development of children with a chronic illness. *Pediatr Clin North Am* **3**: 1–17

Perrin JM, Maclean WE (1988) Children with chronic illness. The prevention of dysfunction. *Pediatr Clini North Am* **35**: 1325–37

Pless IB (1984) Clinical assessment: physical and psychological functioning. *Pediatr Clin North Am* **31**: 33–46

Pless IB, Perrin JM (1985) Issues common to a variety of illnesses. In: Hobbs N, Perrin JM eds. (1985) *Issues in the Care of Children With Chronic Illness*. Jossey Bass, San Francisco

Pless IB, Pinkerton P (1975) *Chronic childhood disorder: promoting patterns of adjustment*. Henry Kempton, London

Renwick R, Brown I, Nagler M (1996) *Quality of life in health promotion and rehabilitation. Conceptual approaches, issues and applications.* Sage Publications, London

Rose MH, Thomas RB (1987) *Children with Chronic Conditions. Nursing in a Family and Community Context.* Grune and Stratton, Ontario

Simmons DP, Jones M, Osborn J, *et al* (1996) Paediatric Rheumatology in the UK: Data from the British Rheumatology Group Register. *Br J Rheumatol* **23**(11): 1975–80

Starfield B (1991) Childhood morbidity: comparisons, clusters and trends. *Pediatrics* **88**(3): 519–26

Stein REK, Jessop DJ (1982) A non categorical approach to chronic childhood illness. *Public Health Rep* **97**: 354–62

Strachan DP, Anderson AR, Limb ES *et al* (1993) A national survey of asthma, prevalence, severity and treatment in Great Britain. *Arch Dis Child* **70**: 174–8

Swartz CL, Hobbie WL, Constine LS *et al* (1994) *Survivors of Childhood Cancer. Assessment and Management.* Mosby, St Louis, Baltimore

Swirydczuk K (1991) Natalia. In: Cooper A, Harper V eds. *This is our child. How parents experience the medical world.* Oxford University Press, Oxford

Thomas RB (1987) In: Rose MH, Thomas RB eds. *Children and Chronic Conditions; Nursing in a Family and Community Context.* Grune Stratton, New York

Thompson RJ, Gustafson KE (1996) *Adaptation to chronic childhood illness.* American Psychological Association, Washington DC

Wiesland SK, Pless IB, Roghman KJ (1992) Chronic illness and mental health problems in pediatric practice. Results from a survey of primary health providers. *Pediatrics* **89**: 445–9

World Health Organisation (1980) *Classification of Impairment, Disability and Handicap.* World Health Organisation, Geneva

Additional quotes obtained through conversations with families. Names have been changed to protect confidentiality. Used with permission.

2

Coping with chronic illness: factors affecting the child's adaptation

Introduction

For all children, childhood is a period of rapid physical, cognitive and emotional development when they face a number of developmental tasks to achieve their optimum growth and development potential. However, development does not occur in a vacuum and all children are significantly influenced by their physical state, psychological competence and the external environment (Vessey and Swanson, 1996). Chronically ill children face the same developmental tasks as 'healthy' children, but mastery of the common tasks and stresses of childhood are made more difficult, as Bradford (1997) suggested,

> '... by the continuing presence of a disease that can significantly alter the child's physical and mental functioning, as well as interactions with the environment.' (p.12)

Thus, in addition to the tasks of childhood, children with chronic illness also face a number of challenges resulting from the diagnosis of a chronic illness.

The consequences of chronic illness for the child

What is it like?

Most discussions about the consequences of chronic illness start from the effects on a child's potential development. Although this discussion will look at such issues it is also important to consider the human element, as sometimes the focus on development does not allow us to understand what it is like from the child's perspective to grow up with a chronic illness.

Children are more aware of what is happening to them than adults perceive. The following extract from the poignant poem, 'I'm still running', by Tracey Wollington who was aged nine years when she was found to have a lymphoma, helps us to understand that consequences are not just objective issues to be evaluated.

> *I can't feel it,*
> *I can't see it,*
> *It's just part of me,*
> *They call it a tumour,*
> *What a name,*
> *No wonder it wants revenge.*

Having a chronic illness is a constant problem and it is important to try to understand the issues from the perspective of the child growing into adulthood. In this way, when exploring the factors that affect the child's development, the issues are related to the individual's needs and are not simply an objective assessment.

Effects of chronic illness

The impact of a chronic illness on the everyday life of a child is difficult to evaluate fully, but these children experience a number of the following consequences of disease which many of their 'healthy' peers do not:

- repeated visits to the doctor or hospital for a 'check up'
- possible repeated admissions to hospital
- repeated extended absences from school
- long-term treatment (drugs, physiotherapy, etc.)
- the distress and discomfort of procedures (blood-taking, bone marrow aspiration, etc.)
- possible unpleasant side effects of treatment (nausea, loss of hair, etc.)
- chronic or continual episodes of pain
- repeated separation from family, friends and school
- restricted activity (isolation due to poor immunity, inability to go out due to treatment, etc.)
- alteration/restriction of diet
- possible threat of death.

These experiences can be stressful and there is an expectation that such stress can both interfere with children's ability to achieve their developmental potential and also cause problems leading to physical and behavioural 'maladaptation' (Stein and Jessop, 1984). Yet, as Eiser (1993) commented:

> *'... the most remarkable finding in all the literature is the extent to which children with chronic disease grow physically and mentally in ways that are largely indistinguishable from the rest of the population.'* (p.16)

The effect of a chronic illness on the development of a child is difficult to predict, as it is not possible to be sure that the failure to meet developmental tasks is due to the chronic illness alone. Clearly there is no way of knowing what other factors would have affected the development of the child if the disease had been absent, but the consequences of a chronic illness may create a barrier and limit a child's ability to achieve a developmental task.

Chronic illness and child development

Frameworks of assessment

Most studies exploring the impact of chronic illness utilise the theoretical frameworks, for example Piaget (1929, 1952) for cognitive; Erickson (1959, 1963) for personal-social; and Kohlberg (1969) for moral development. These models are built on the assumption that certain developmental tasks need to be obtained within a certain age range. Development occurs through maturity and experience, and as children achieve a task they move on to a more advanced developmental level (Cerreto, 1986). There has been some criticism of the linear approach to development as it fails to address how children move from one stage to another, or to acknowledge the impact of past experience, culture and social environment on a child's development (Nelson, 1986). However, this approach continues to be widely used in research and practice as it offers a framework to evaluate a child's progress.

Incomplete data on chronic illness

A number of authors (Eiser, 1993; Bradford, 1997; Whyte, 1997) have acknowledged that the emotional and practical consequences of a chronic disorder will vary according to the child's developmental level. However, this has been difficult to support empirically due to the incomplete data available for chronic illness across all age ranges. Some conditions are diagnosed within a certain age range (for example, epilepsy onset is usually between five and seven years) so the research available doesn't cover all age groups for all conditions. However, even where the incidence is more evenly spread, such as in asthma, it is difficult to use measures across all age groups.

Due to the incomplete data, our understanding of the impact of chronic illness on a child at different developmental stages is largely theoretical. Thus the framework is based on inferences drawn from models used to describe children's expected developmental 'norms'. The processes and events (which can be physical, psychological or environmental) that interfere with the normal sequences can disrupt the attainment of a developmental task (Bradford, 1997). Chronic illness, by modifying the maturation and experiences of the child, has the potential to make developmental tasks more difficult to achieve.

Assessment of development

There is a tendency to assume that chronic illness has a negative effect on development, whereas some research has suggested that illness and disability may have some positive effects on adjustment and personality development (Gliedman and Roth, 1980; Drotar *et al*, 1981). It is important not to automatically label these children as developmentally delayed as a child may achieve the tasks appropriate for their age (Kazack, 1989). What is clear is that chronic illness is a variable that can influence the development of children, and there is a need to make sure that any negative effects are minimised thus ensuring that children reach their optimum developmental potential.

Factors influencing development.

It is difficult to predict the impact of chronic illness on development as the characteristics of the disease, child, family and society vary and these factors interact, acting as a kind of feedback loop (see *Figure 2.1*).

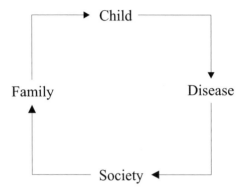

Figure 2.1: Feedback loop illustrating the interrelationship of chronic disease, child and family

As Perrin and Gerrity (1984) stated:

> *'... the illness affects the individual's interactions with the physical and social environment in which he or she lives, and aspects of the child's environment such as parents, peers or school systems are altered as a result of the illness.'* (p.841)

Characteristics of the disease

The features of chronic illness, as a broad category, which may affect the child's ability to cope with the problems and achieve developmental milestones, can vary enormously. It is important to appreciate that the characteristics of the disease in themselves do not indicate the degree of adjustment or developmental delay, as this can also be influenced by the child's and/or the family's perception of the degree of severity and limitations of the disorder. However, developmental delay may be influenced by the following:

- *degree of physical handicap:* The risk of developmental delay increases with the severity of physical handicap. This limits the child's ability to perform developmental tasks. Cadman *et al*

(1987) found that children with a chronic illness and physical disability were three times more at risk of psychiatric disorder when compared to their 'healthy' peers

- *problems of bowel/bladder control:* Incontinence problems such as 'soiling' can create embarrassing odours for children and can affect acceptance of children by their peers
- *degree of mental disability:* This can interfere with the ability to achieve developmental milestones
- *severity and duration of the illness:* Repeated admissions to hospital or ongoing treatments can interrupt education and the development of peer relationships
- *degree of difference or changes to the appearance:* This can affect acceptance and degree of participation in group activities (Turner-Henson *et al*, 1994)
- *unpredictable nature of the disorder:* Children who suffer from disorders with unpredictable problems, such as epileptic fits, may suffer fear, and isolation from social activities (Austin, 1996).

Characteristics of the child

The individual characteristics of a child can affect the ability of that child to cope with the consequences of chronic illness. Some relevant factors include:

- *age at diagnosis/stage of development:* The limitations imposed by chronic illness have different implications for the tasks to be achieved for each age group
- *gender:* There are different expectations of children's behaviour which may affect the way they cope with stressful situations. The study by Eiser *et al* (1992) gives support to the data that parents' appraisal of adjustment or restrictions are indicators of a child's adjustment, and perceptions of gender-appropriate coping behaviours may be modelled by the parents
- *personality/temperament:* Children with chronic illnesses display the same variety of individual differences as children without chronic illness. Some traits, such as temperament, are present at birth whereas others, such as self-concept, develop over time. A strong self-concept is developed through the mastery of physical, intellectual, social and emotional tasks which means that children with multiple problems are at increased risk of developmental delay (Newacheck and Stoddard, 1994)

- *coping styles:* Much of the research on children's coping has focused on evaluating their distress during medical procedures. Findings by Bryng-Hall (1995) suggest that children who feel secure and have parents who demonstrate a positive discipline style are able to cope 'better' with distressing experiences.

Characteristics of the family

The ability of children to 'cope' cannot be evaluated in isolation as it is the way in which their families handle the difficulties that influences their behaviour. A number of factors have been noted as affecting children's coping skills:

- *marriage stability:* Families who demonstrated open communication and a sharing of responsibilities had a positive influence on the children's and families' ability to cope with the effects of the chronic illness (Clawson, 1996)
- *family resources:* Financial, physical, emotional and social networks enable families to 'cope' with the demands of children with a chronic illness
- *social background:* The social and cultural background influences attitudes and practices with regard to the management of the demands of care and the provision of networks of support
- *parenting styles:* Parents' management style has been recognised as a contributory factor in children's adaptation to chronic illness (Knafl *et al*, 1996).

Characteristics of society

The effect of chronic illness is not merely a response of the child and family, for the ability to cope with chronic illness is shaped and influenced by the values of the society in which it occurs (Turner-Henson *et al*, 1994). Society's reactions to children and families with a chronic illness affect the ways families cope with the problems of the disease and feelings of 'being different'. For example:

- experiences of stigma can result in feelings of isolation (Gray, 1993)
- 'unacceptable' behaviour is evaluated by society's expectations of 'normal' development and behaviour within each age group, and

'inappropriate' behaviour can be a source of embarrassment for the family (Gray, 1993)
* prejudice/discrimination in the allocation and accessibility of resources that can affect the family's ability to cope practically and emotionally with the demands of chronic illness.

Consequences of chronic illness

Stein and Jessop (1988) suggested that chronic illness at the time of diagnosis or as the illness progressed would produce one or more of the following problems:

* limitation of ability to perform tasks appropriate to the child's age and development
* disfigurement
* dependency on medication and/or special diet to control symptoms
* dependency on technology (such as ventilators, infusion pumps)
* the need for medical care and/or support services in addition to requirements for the child's age
* special ongoing treatments at home or at school.

Such consequences can affect every aspect of life for the child and family. Care can become more time-consuming and complicated as the child has to adjust to new diets, drugs and procedures which have to be integrated into everyday life. These changes have both practical and emotional implications, as 'normal' child-rearing practices can take on a new perspective for the child and family.

Summary

1   The impact of chronic illness on children is difficult to evaluate fully, but there are a number of consequences that their 'healthy' peers do not experience, such as repeated illness, hospitalisation, medications and alterations or restrictions to their diet.

2   How a child copes with the changes is influenced by:
    * the severity and degree of disability as a result of the disease
    * the child's coping style
    * the child's developmental level

- the family's ability to adapt to the changes
- society's attitudes to the disorder.

All these factors can affect the child's ability to achieve their growth and development potential.

Implications for practice

The aim of care is to foster an environment that enables children to achieve their growth and development potential. Thus it is important for practitioners to do the following:

1 To gain an understanding of the impact of those factors that influence a child's and family's adaptation to chronic illness from the child's and family's perspective.

2 To utilise this knowledge when assessing each family, in order to identify the factors that may affect, aid or hinder each child's and family's adaptation to chronic illness.

3 To explore the consequences of chronic illness and treatment with each family, to ensure negotiated management strategies which will positively influence child and family and enable the child to achieve both growth and development potential.

References

Austin JK (1996) A model of family adaptation to new onset childhood epilepsy. *J Neurosci Nurs* **26**(2): 82–92

Bradford R (1997) *Children, families and chronic disease. Psychological models and methods of care.* Routledge Publications, London

Bryng-Hall J (1995) *Rewriting family scripts.* Guilford Press, London

Cadman D, Boyle M, Szatmari P, *et al* (1987) Chronic illness, disability and mental and social well being. Findings of the Ontario Child Health Survey. *Pediatrics* **79**: 705–12

Cerreto MC (1986) Developmental issues in chronic illness: implications and applications. *Topics in Early Childhood Special Education* **5**(4): 23–35

Clawson JA (1996) A child with chronic illness and the process of family adaptation. *J Pediatr Nurs* **11**(1): 52–61

Drotar D, Doershuck F, Stern RC *et al* (1981) Psychosocial functioning of children with cystic fibrosis. *Pediatrics* **67**: 338–43

Eiser C, Havermans T, Pancer M *et al* (1992) Adjustment to chronic disease in relation to age, and gender: mothers' and fathers' reports of their children's behaviour. *J Pediatr Psychol* **17**(3): 261–75

Eiser C (1993) *Growing up with a chronic disease. The impact on children and their families.* Jessica Kingsley Publications, London

Erickson EH (1959) Identity and the life cycle. *Psychol Issues* **1**: 18–164

Erickson EH (1963) *Childhood and Society.* Norton, New York

Gliedman J, Roth W (1980) *The Unexpected Minority: Handicapped Children in America. Prepared for the Carnegie Council on Children.* Harcourt Brace Jovanovich, New York

Gray DE (1993) Perceptions of stigma; parents of autistic children. *Sociol Health Illness* **15**(1): 103–20

Jessop DJ, Stein RK (1988) Essential concepts in the care of children with chronic illness. *Pediatrics* **15**: 5–12

Kazack AE (1989) Families of chronically ill children: A systems and social-ecological model of adaptation and coping. *J Consult Clin Psychol* **57**: 25–30

Kohlberg L (1969) Stage and sequence: the cognitive-developmental analysis of children's sex role concepts and attitudes. In: Goslin D ed. *Handbook of Socialization Theory and Research.* Rand McNally, Chicago

Knafl K, Brietmaer B, Gallo A, *et al* (1996) Family responses to childhood chronic illness: description of management styles. *J Pediatr Nurs* **11**(5): 315–26

Nelson K (1986) *Event Knowledge: Structure and Function in Development.* Lawrence Erlbaum, New Jersey

Newacheck PW, Stoddard JJ (1994) Prevalence and impact of multiple chronic childhood illnesses. *J Pediatr* **124**: 40–8

Perrin EC, Gerritty PS (1984) Development of children with chronic illness. *Pediatrics* **67**: 841–9

Piaget J (1929) *The Child's Conception of the World.* Harcourt Brace Jovanovich, New York

Piaget J (1952) *The origins of intelligence in children.* International University Press, New York

Stein REK, Jessop DJ (1984) Psychological adjustment among children with chronic conditions. *Pediatrics* **73**: 169–74

Turner-Henson A, Holaday B, Ogletree G *et al* (1994) The experiences of discrimination: challenges for chronically ill children. *Pediatr Nurs* **20**(6): 571–7

Vessey JA, Swanson MN (1996) Chronic Conditions and Child Development. In: Jackson P (1996) *Primary Care of the Child With a Chronic Condition.* 2nd edn. Mosby, St Louis

Whyte DA (1997) *Explorations in Family Nursing.* Routledge, London

Wollington T (1990) I'm still running. In: Baum JD, Dominica Sister F, Woodward RN (1990) *Listen. My Child Has a Lot of Living to Do.* Oxford University Press, Oxford

Additional quotes obtained through conversations with families. Names have been changed to protect confidentiality. Used with permission.

3
Chronic illness and development: the effects on children's developmental stages

Introduction

As Patterson (1988) stated:

> *'For the chronically ill child, the normative psychosocial and cognitive tasks of development interact with the hardships of the illness repeatedly throughout the child's life.'* (p.82)

Childhood chronic illness takes on new meanings as the child grows and develops. The child and family face the challenge of how best to meet the child's needs at a given age within the limitations of the illness. The limitations of many chronic illnesses shape development from infancy to adolescence, making the achievement of tasks difficult and sometimes impossible. Thus, it is essential to evaluate the potential impact of chronic illness on normal developmental expectations and to explore ways of minimising the problems and enabling children to reach their potential.

Children's development

Infancy (0–2 years)

The hallmark of infancy is the egocentric inability to differentiate between the self and the world. Infants spend their first eighteen months in a dependency relationship with adults as they learn about themselves and the world around them. The focus of research in infancy has been on the parent-child attachment process, as the quality of this relationship is seen as central to the future achievement of developmental milestones. Park and Waters (1989) found, at least with healthy infants, that more securely attached infants appeared to be more sociable with peers and unfamiliar adults at one year of age.

According to the attachment theory, the development of a primary social attachment is the main task of infancy (Bowlby, 1969). As Cerreto (1986) stated:

> *'Infants must establish trust in others to meet their basic needs, develop emotional ties, experience and master stranger anxiety and develop the beginnings of a sense of intentionality of their own acts.'* (p.25)

Attachment

Chronic illness can affect the process of bonding between the parents and the infant and so can undermine the way in which the parents foster healthy psycho-social development. Much of the work has concentrated on the mother-infant relationship, as the mother often spends most time with the infant. Factors which appear to interfere with the attachment process include:

- the disease process and treatments interfering with the 'normal' interaction between the mother and infant
- demands of care leaving little time for affection
- guilt about causes of the infant's illness
- uncertainty about the prognosis of the disease.

Having a child with a chronic illness and an uncertain future, makes the bonding process difficult. This is illustrated by the following extract showing the mother's uncertainty and her difficulty in accepting her child:

> *'We need to find a name for "it". I look at our newborn baby with the old, old face and feel it already has a name; we have to guess what it is. If we guess wrongly it dies... . Deep inside me, I acknowledge I don't want to give a favourite name to a child who will die.'* (p.14)
>
> (Hilary Barrett [1991] about Jackie who was born prematurely)

There is also the issue of the quality of the mothering and, as a research study by Goldberg *et al* (1990) indicated, secure attachments are found in those mothers who are more attentive to, and able to anticipate the needs of, their infants. The process of how chronic illness affects the quality of the attachment between the mother and the infant is not clearly understood, although a study by Linde *et al* (1966) found that children who had been wrongly diagnosed to have heart conditions were found to be more restricted in their activities when they were compared to healthy children. It seems that the beliefs about the child's problems may be a greater determinant of the interaction than the disorder itself.

Sensorimotor discrimination

Parents need to foster a sense of trust and promote development through nurturing, touch and sensory stimulation of the infant (Cerreto, 1986). The infant learns to understand the world through interaction with objects; according to how they look, feel and taste. Thus a child with a sensory impairment, a condition that is physically limiting and/or painful, or an environment that reduces or modifies sensory experiences (such as an incubator), is at risk of having a distorted view of the world and a less secure attachment to a central caregiver.

The development of trust in early infancy depends on experiences that meet the infants' needs on time and in an appropriate manner. So, an infant cries and a caregiver feeds, changes or soothes the infant. Trust in a central caregiver and his or her ability to make things happen to meet the infant's needs is likely to produce a secure infant. This requires a continuous relationship with a primary caregiver. However, the attachment process may be interrupted when an infant goes through extended periods of illness or hospitalisation.

Hospitalisation

The hospitalised infant will experience separation from parents, painful procedures and interaction with a variety of strangers. However, the impact of the hospital environment on the infant's development is difficult to evaluate. A number of studies have explored both the quality of the environment as a factor that may influence sensory stimulation and the possible implications this may have on the development of the infant (Wells *et al*, 1994). An infant who is ventilated, in an incubator, having enteral or intravenous feeding, with touching minimised to procedures and treatment due to the child's condition, has a distorted interaction with parents and the environment. This affects the parents' ability to identify with their child, as Hilary Barrett so sadly comments:

> *'From the first minutes of her birth, Jackie was surrounded by machines, drips, wires, tubes. By the second day of her life she was under ultraviolet lights... her face looked like a lizard's or a frog's, not like that of a human baby.'* (p.17)

Thus, not only may ill infants have very limited experience of secure comforting, such as when their mothers cuddle them or provide food to reduce feelings of hunger, but also the parents do not always have the opportunity for 'normal' parenting experiences which would enhance bonding and secure attachment.

The difficulty of bonding may continue long after the initial hospitalisation as parents continue to feel anxiety due to the illness, continued treatment and possible readmission to hospital. Under such circumstances, it can prove difficult to form attachments with the infants as they may have problems feeding, have interrupted sleep and be difficult to comfort due to pain or the presence of technology such as feeding tubes or infusions. Any or all of these factors may contribute to the behaviour of the infant and the response of parents in the bonding process. As Lester and Zeskind (1979) noted, premature babies have higher, more urgent cries than their healthy counterparts and this, in turn, can create stress, with parents becoming exhausted and finding it difficult to offer comforting experiences beyond the requirements of treatment and essential care. To what extent a primary caregiver can compensate for interruptions to the bonding process is difficult to evaluate empirically, but secure attachment to a primary caregiver has been shown to be an important element in enabling infants to achieve their development potential (Cerreto, 1986).

Summary

1 Infants require the presence of a central caregiver to provide comfort and nurturing, and to promote a secure attachment which will facilitate future development.

2 As a result of illness, periods of hospitalisation and ongoing treatment, chronic illness can interfere with bonding by distorting the experiences of the parents and the infant.

Toddlerhood (2–3 years)

This is a period of significant milestones for children as they gain a number of important skills, such as walking, talking and control of bodily elimination. It can be a very exciting time for the parents of healthy children but a most stressful period for the parents of sick and disabled children as there is an increasing awareness that the children are not gaining the skills appropriate to their age, or are doing so at a much slower rate than their peers (Wasserman and Allen, 1985).

The emergence of an ability to symbolise thought processes into language marks the end of infancy and the beginning of toddlerhood (Cerretto, 1986). The child begins to use imagery and memory and to develop a degree of self-reliance, but at the same time remains very vulnerable. It is a period of exploration as toddlers begin to assert themselves and test the limits of adult control, though at this stage children may not cope well with separation. It is a time when the child begins to learn control and autonomy and it can be an uncertain period leading to shame and insecurity for the child if not handled properly (Erickson, 1959, 1964).

Autonomy verses shame

Coping with the challenge of toddlers has been noted as one of the most stressful periods for parents as the children learn to assert themselves. This is a period of upheaval when toddlers express their own wishes regardless of others, resorting to tantrums and stubbornness as they seek to gain their own way. Even simple tasks, such as dressing and eating, can become a battle of wits. However, the child remains vulnerable and still needs the security and comfort of the parents. Finding the right balance can be a difficult process for the parents of 'healthy' children, and faced with the additional problems of chronic illness, further strain can be added to family life as the parents try to ensure that their child receives a particular treatment to manage the symptoms of a chronic illness. As one mother noted:

> *'Rich went through a bad patch and I couldn't get him to do anything. I couldn't get him to take his enzymes and he would hide under the table every time physio was due. I felt terrible — as if it was my fault — I mean, it was my responsibility... [laughs]... sometimes it took all morning to get through everything... my husband will tell you... it was my job and the house was a tip.'*

(Mum about Richard, aged 3 years)

Given the toddler's normal developmental drive for independence from parents, the presence of a chronic illness can fuel the parent-child conflict typical of this age.

Skills development

A large part of a toddler's drive for autonomy and self-control is through the active exploration of the environment. Self-mastery of their newly emerging gross motor skills, together with external encouragement of normal activities in toddlers will promote normal growth and development. Yet the realities of the restrictions of the chronic disease may mean that these children are unable to explore the limits of their environment actively due to disability or tiredness, and tasks become more difficult to achieve. For example, toilet training — important in the development of self-control — is hindered by the inability to sit for any length of time or becomes less pleasurable due to the presence of foul-smelling stools in chronic conditions such as cystic fibrosis (Frauman and Brandon, 1996).

Parents may find it difficult to give a child autonomy. Indeed, they may discourage them from actively pursuing goals and encourage a passive approach due to feelings of guilt or over-protectiveness and concerns that include:

- exposure to environmental hazards (eg. allergens in asthma)
- fear of exposure to negative experiences from other children (eg. taunts about loss of hair due to chemotherapy)
- fear of injury (eg. sustained bleeding in haemophilia)
- the need to ensure treatments are given which the child doesn't want or like (eg. physiotherapy for cystic fibrosis).

These restrictions reduce the opportunity for practising the skills of self-expression and self-control, and can also slow the attainment of mastery of the physical skills of elimination control, walking and talking.

Parent-toddler interaction

There is an assumption in literature on the subject, that the presence of chronic illness in some way distorts the interaction between the toddler and parents which, in turn, influences the developmental progress of the toddler. The focus in research has been the parent-child interaction, with the aim of measuring the differences in play and communication processes (Bradford, 1997). However, the findings indicated few differences in the way parents interacted with the child compared to the parents of their 'healthy' counterparts, but it was noted that chronically ill children were more passive and compliant. Yet, as Eiser (1993) noted:

> *'Future work needs to untangle whether this can be attributed to differences in parenting, or is a response to hospitalisation, intrusions from treatment and separations from the normal family life.'* (p.41)

All intrusions in a toddler's life may be viewed as potentially stressful, and chronic illness can be identified as a potential source of stress and insecurity.

Regression

Managing the care of a chronically ill toddler, with their behavioural and temperamental characteristics, reliance on routines and limited ability to communicate their thoughts and feelings verbally, can make it difficult to cope with the additional stresses of chronic illness (Garrison and McQuiston, 1989) and the subsequent treatment and hospitalisation. Given the difficulty of gaining information from the toddler, research has tended to focus on parents' — and largely mothers' — perceptions of their children. Wysoki *et al* (1989) emphasised that mothers reported anxiety, depression, sleep and appetite problems in toddlers who 'internalised' the stress of the restrictions of diabetes management. It may be that these reactions are no different for toddlers without diabetes, and that toddlers may demonstrate this behaviour when faced with a stressful event. However, the research findings serve to highlight the effects of stress and the potential impact of chronic illness on the toddler. Although the impact of the stress of chronic illness is difficult to evaluate, and loss of previously achieved tasks (behavioural regression) has been documented as a consequence of hospitalisation and treatment in children of all ages, it is, however, most commonly noted in this age group (Vessey and Swanson, 1996).

Summary

1 Toddlerhood is a period during which there is a significant development of such skills as walking, talking and control of

bodily elimination. Chronic illness can affect the attainment of these skills.

2   Chronic illness is a source of stress for the toddler due to illness and periods of hospitalisation, when the toddler may not cope well with separation.

3   The balance between allowing the toddler autonomy and ensuring treatments for chronic illness is a difficult one for parents and can fuel the conflicts typical of this age.

Pre-school (4–5 years)

The pre-school stage has been described as a period of 'relative calm' (Eiser, 1993) after the turmoil of toddlerhood, but there are a number of important developmental tasks that need to be achieved prior to the child beginning school. The central task of pre-school children is to put their newly-established sense of autonomy to work actively, for example by investigating the environment outside the home when attending a nursery. Other children begin school early through reception classes.

The pre-school child is developing physically and cognitively to achieve the skills of independence and exploration (Cerretto, 1986), and for many children this is a time when they begin to develop social skills through relationships outside the family. But these children, although becoming increasingly independent, are still vulnerable and while they are able to plan and carry out activities, in doing so they may 'go too far' and feel guilty about the outcome (Patterson, 1988).

Learning rules

This is an active period of social and physical development when pre-school children actively engage in play in order to learn about their ever-expanding world. Key tasks for the pre-school child are to learn cultural rules, expectations of right and wrong, and sex roles. Play activities are often centred around discovering and testing these rules. Pre-school children are still fairly egocentric and can become more assertive and aggressive as they develop initiative and curiosity. The child tests and evaluates the order and relationship of rules which can result in frequent cries of 'It's not fair!' at this stage. The development of initiative and curiosity runs parallel to the testing of limits, but pre-school children are still vulnerable to guilt and feelings of shame

(Erickson, 1959, 1964) and they need adults to set clear limits, provide protection and foster a sense of control, power and competence to produce a sense of achievement (Cerreto, 1986; Patterson, 1988). Setting clear limits to behaviour may prove problematic when a child has a chronic illness and goes through periods of acute exacerbation of the condition, or hospitalisation. Expectations and discipline may need to be modified according to the child's condition and this can send mixed messages of what is acceptable behaviour to the child.

Social development

Social development through opportunities is an important feature of pre-school development, but the restrictions of a chronic illness may limit the social interaction of the pre-school child with a chronic condition. Restrictions may be due to a lack of physical development, stamina or the effects of treatment and can limit a child's contribution in both play activities and contact with others, thereby reducing opportunities for the development of social skills.

A key task in the pre-school child's development of social skills is learning to adapt to the expectations of others. There is a move away from egocentric behaviour and a desire to please others, as well as a developing of relationships with peers and other adults. However, for children with a chronic illness, this may also be a time when they gain their first awareness of 'being different' (Anderson, 1995) and this may affect their interaction with others when trying to 'fit in'.

Body concept

The physical tasks of the pre-school child involve the refinement of general body and fine muscle control. The developmental stage related tasks involve developing and refining an adequate body concept and an understanding about sex differences. A child with a chronic illness may have difficulty in formulating a healthy body image particularly if most of their awareness is associated with disability and discomfort (Vessey and Swanson, 1996). Pre-school children are emotionally very vulnerable and nightmares, phobias and the fear of loss of a body part are typical of this age (Patterson, 1988). Thus, when treatment requires surgery or invasive procedures it can contribute to a feeling of insecurity and loss of control which may, in turn, affect a child's self-esteem and body image.

Beliefs about illness

Intellectually pre-school children are at the pre-operational stage (Piaget, 1929, 1952) where they centre on concrete aspects of their experience. At this stage children can assume that experiences are a result of something they did (Bibbace and Walsh, 1980). They have a correlational, rather than a causal, approach to understanding which means they are likely to assume that the illness is because of something they did. For example, they might think that an asthma attack had been brought on by 'breathing too fast'. Such children often describe the cause of the illness in terms of a sight or sound which may bear no relation to it's actual cause. Cerretto (1986) illustrates this point:

> *'Why do you have diabetes? "From drinking too much water before bed." How did drinking too much water before bed make you have diabetes? "Too much water before bed makes you sick."'* (p.29)

Such misconceptions, together with the preoccupation with winning approval, can lead to beliefs that a cure for their illness can be achieved by following the rules (Perrin and Gerrity, 1984). Such beliefs may lead to inappropriate behaviour and reduced motivation in moving on to the next developmental stage.

Summary

1 The important and central tasks of the pre-school child are to develop independence, to learn cultural rules and to develop social relationships.

2 Chronic illness can adversely affect the child's ability to 'fit in' and repeated episodes of illness and hospitalisation can limit social interaction.

3 Pre-school children are vulnerable to phobias and nightmares and chronic illness can contribute to feelings of insecurity and misconceptions about illness and treatment.

School age (6–11 years)

Acquiring a sense of accomplishment through skill development and sustained effort is a central task of 'middle childhood' (Erickson, 1959, 1964). During this period children form close relationships with other children of the same sex and develop new intellectual, athletic and artistic skills. The child develops self-esteem primarily through the achievement of these skills, and approval through peer relationships which provides a sense of identity and belonging (Kelner, 1995).

The importance of attending school in achieving the tasks of school-age children has been stressed by a number of authors (Wietzman, 1984; Norton-Fowler *et al*, 1985) as the way for the child to develop social relationships outside their family. Academic achievement, regular attendance and social competence are major goals during this developmental period.

School attendance

As Eiser (1993) noted:

> *'The importance of school for children should not be underestimated... as it is often the "yardstick" by which the impact of the disease is assessed.'* (p.46)

It is considered advantageous for a child to return to school after an absence as it provides an opportunity for both child and family to achieve some sort of 'normal life' routine by allowing parents to return to work and the child to continue with their academic and social development. As one mother commented:

> *'It was hard — all those months of treatment. I never thought it would end, although I didn't think about that at the time. I just wanted him better and I was prepared to do anything... but my whole life was wrapped up in visiting the hospital. You know, it wasn't until Steven went back to school and I got a part-time job that I realised other people had been getting on with their lives. It was strange not going to the hospital... it was great to have some sort of life... I don't know how I did it. I suppose you just do.'*

(Mum talking about Steven, aged 7, after chemotherapy for cancer)

However, in practice such children may find both attendance and achievement at school problematic due to the following factors:

- repeated absence as a result of periods of illness, attendance for outpatient treatments and hospital admission
- missed lessons creating the disadvantages of such problems as 'catching up' academically and re-establishing relationships with peers
- rejection by peers due to illness and consequences of treatment, for example loss of hair due to chemotherapy
- restrictions imposed by the disorder and treatment, for example the breathlessness of cystic fibrosis limits participation in athletic activities and the required physiotherapy can take the child away from other activities during the day
- compromised intellectual and behavioural abilities due to the effects of the disease and its treatment
- protective parents keeping the child from school to reduce the impact of rejection or failure on the child.

Even if there is no significant absence from school, aspects of the disorder such as dietary or medication needs and time away from their peers for treatments during the day, can serve to set children with chronic illness apart from their peers. These interruptions can single out a child as 'different' and have an impact on the child's willingness to return to school. Although the literature indicates that children with cancer have been documented as having 'extreme school phobia' (Eiser, 1980, 1993) this does not appear to be the case for other disorders, although the research on other chronic illnesses is limited. However, it is not surprising that there is evidence of extended school absence due to illness for children with chronic illness and this can affect their academic achievement, their ability to keep pace with their peers and hence their ability to achieve developmental goals.

Academic achievement

Perceptions about a school-age child's academic ability and misunderstandings about chronic illness can lead to unrealistic expectations of a child's potential. Patterson (1988) cites a number of studies which have found significantly lower academic achievement among selected groups of chronically ill children with normal cognitive ability. Although children's underachievement may be a feature of poor school attendance, Eiser and Town (1987) found that there was a lack of understanding about chronic illness amongst teachers, with both an uncertainty of how to manage the child's condition and the holding of inappropriate stereotypes which could also affect expectations of the child's development. Low expectations of academic achievement for a child with chronic illness may lead to consistent underachievement, compromising the child's sense of competence and mastery of developmental tasks.

The effects of school absence, chronic illness and treatment can make success at school harder to achieve, which in turn can contribute to a lack of self-esteem and affect the way children interact with their peers. Chronically ill children who lack confidence or the skills to integrate with their peers may remain socially isolated and have an increased risk of emotional problems.

Social development

Involvement with and acceptance by the peer group at this age is important to social development and children will worry about their differences. 'Healthy' children can struggle with their need for acceptance and other children can single out small differences to tease a 'different' child. Differences such as diet, medication or treatments can be used to taunt a child resulting in withdrawal from social situations either by the child fearful of rejection or by parents in an effort to prevent the child from emotional damage. For whatever reason, any withdrawal makes it much more difficult for the child to develop social skills and gain independence from the family.

Brietmayer *et al* (1992) found in a study of 7 to14 year olds that children with chronic illness were at an increased risk of 20 to 30 per cent for social competence difficulties when compared to their 'healthy' counterparts. However, families are a key element in developing social skills, and the children of families who enabled them to develop strategies to deal with the alterations in social relationships as a result of chronic illness were more able to cope, which in turn prevented potential difficulties.

Hospitalisation

School-age children need a sense of control over their environment through sustained effort. Children with chronic illness who have repeated bouts of illness or hospitalisation may feel powerless and this may affect their development, given the need for this age group to have a sense of mastery over situations.

School-age children are in the concrete operational stage of psychological development (Piaget, 1929, 1952) where they view illness in terms of germs or contamination (Bibbace and Walsh, 1980; Perrin and Gerritty, 1984) and may believe that by following instructions they can cure their illness. The ongoing nature of chronic illness can therefore be difficult for children of this age to understand.

Summary

1   Acquiring a sense of achievement through sustained effort is the central task of middle childhood.

2   School attendance for academic achievement and social development is important but may be difficult due to the effects of chronic illness.

3   Repeated 'bouts' of hospitalisation are particularly difficult to cope with at this age, given the children's need for mastery over situations.

Adolescence (12–16 years)

Adolescence is an exciting time of transition with major physiological, psychological and social changes. The main developmental task for the adolescent is to discover and establish an independent adult identity (Erickson 1959, 1964). Yet, as Marcia (1982) noted:

> '... if the termination of adolescence were to depend on the formation of an identity, then, for some, it would never end.' (p.159)

Adolescence has become associated with the task of acquiring an identity — something we all go through in our lives. So, although this developmental process is distinctive in adolescence, it is not exclusive to it. However, there are a number of physical and psychosocial adjustments the adolescent needs to go through.

Physically, adolescence begins with the emergence of the secondary sexual characteristics and ends with the emergence of an adult identity, although as we have already established there is no clear-cut ending to this development (Manworren, 1996). Society's perception of adult status varies between cultures, and in western society the law doesn't decree a single age to indicate adult status in all aspects of life, as illustrated by the various ages at which an individual can legally marry (16 years), hold a driving licence (17 years) and vote (18 years).

This 'process' of adolescence is about the mastery of a number of key tasks required to be able to function independently in society (Yoos, 1987). These tasks include:

• developing a comfortable body image
• building an identity through socialisation
• the establishment of meaningful relationships
• forming a sexual identity
• establishing economic and emotional independence.

Adolescence is a period of immense change which has, in the past, been characterised as a period of 'storm and stress' when adolescents try to assert their own independent identity separate from their parents. However, this approach exaggerated the nature of adolescence and, although some individuals may have problems, the generalisation to all adolescents as potential troublemakers with problems tended to create a stereotyped approach to understanding the process of development.

Traditional theories that emerged from this 'storm and stress' perspective attached special importance to the parent–adolescent conflict, laying emphasis on early separation from parents to foster healthy development. However, more recent research (Irwin, 1987) has found that early separation has a negative effect on the development of the adolescent who can feel vulnerable and unsupported as a result. Thus there is a general acceptance that adolescence is not inherently turbulent and the emphasis is now on fostering healthy development through family strategies that renegotiate the responsibilities and obligations of the adolescent as they go through this period of transition (Baumrind, 1987). Parenting styles that have open communication, flexibility and consistent support but firm enforcement of clear rules, have been cited as having a positive influence on adolescents' ego development and a reduction in their vulnerability to peer pressure (Hauser, 1991).

Physiological changes

The adolescent goes through a number of physiological changes including an increase in body mass, changing muscle proportions and the development of secondary sex characteristics. All of these changes contribute to the development of a good body image, self-esteem and the formation of an identity. However, the presence of a chronic illness can interfere with 'normal' physiological processes.

Physiological changes may interact directly with the symptoms of the disease, as in the case of diabetes where increasing hormonal changes and neuroregulators lead to increases in blood sugar levels despite strict adherence to the diet and injections of insulin (Anderson, 1995). The effects of these physiological changes can serve to undermine the adolescent's efforts at self-care and reduce their willingness to comply with treatment (Baumrind, 1987; Anderson, 1995). In some cases, the presence of a chronic disease can slow normal physiological processes and delay growth spurts.

Yoos (1987) stresses that adolescents are normally preoccupied with their rapidly-developing bodily functions and changes as they acquire an individual body image. Body image is a dynamic process which is influenced by both 'normal' adolescent development and society's expectations. Thus, some chronically ill adolescents may have a poor body image and identity formation, as disability or body disfigurement reduce their ability to participate in group activities and further aggravate the 'normal' adolescent concerns of being physically attractive and accepted.

Identity

For chronically ill adolescents, identity means not only discovering their own personality, values, beliefs and career choices, but also discovering the reality of their illness and the resulting limitations that may be placed on their progression into such adult roles as getting a job and having a family. As Suzanne Armour commented:

> *'Andrew knows a great deal about his illness. He has learnt to accept the fact his adolescent growth spurt is likely to be long delayed and he has been outstripped long ago by his peer group with their big feet, great height, and breaking voices, while he still looks about 12 years old. He has learnt to accept he will never have children. He has learnt to accept the different aspects of his treatment, some of which are not pleasant. He has to face a future of very uncertain health. Greatest of all he has to accept his own mortality over the last few years as he watched children he has known well with*

*CF deteriorate in health and then learned of their deaths.
None of this has been easy or exactly "normal".'*

(Armour, 1991)

Concerns about physical attractiveness, sexuality and reproductive competence are particularly troubling for many adolescents. The added complications of chronic illness, particularly if the problem is visible, can interfere with sexual expression and contribute to feelings of inadequacy. Although all adolescents engage in such activities as dieting to improve their body image, it has been shown that adolescents with a chronic illness, across a number of chronic conditions, have higher body dissatisfaction and engage in more high-risk strategies to lose weight than their 'healthy' counterparts (Neumark-Steiner *et al*, 1995). This has implications for controlling the symptoms of such chronic illnesses as diabetes where diet plays an important role in maintaining health and preventing complications, and interference in symptom control creates a cascade of ongoing physical problems which can add to the individual's feelings of poor body image and self-esteem.

Decreasing dependence

The general expectation that adolescents should be gaining a degree of separation from their parents can be a difficult one for children with chronic illness. For many, chronic illness makes it difficult to achieve independence particularly when they need others to provide some aspects of their care and treatment. Although the adolescent can often take control over parts of treatment such as taking medication, where there are disabilities the burden of care still falls to the parents or other family members and this can create worries about how the adolescent will be able to leave home and gain independence. The transition of care from families to others or to the adolescents themselves is a difficult one, with some families prolonging dependence due to the unpredictability of certain conditions, such as hypoglycaemia in diabetes; exacerbations of the chronic illness and episodes of acute illness being not uncommon at this stage (Patterson, 1988).

The search for an independent identity, with adolescents striving to make decisions for themselves, may be difficult given the realities of the illness, and anger and rebellion may be the result. Indeed, non-compliance in such instances may be utilised by adolescents as a way of taking control of their own care.

Adolescent concerns

It is difficult to evaluate the concerns of chronically ill adolescents although Dragone (1990) constructed a health risk questionnaire with a small group of them. This highlighted that chronically ill adolescents had similar concerns to their 'healthy' peers, such as being unable to meet with friends, acne and being overweight. However, the experience of a chronic illness adds to such concerns and sets the adolescent apart. Being aware of a lifelong illness can make adolescents feel more vulnerable and that, together with the limitations imposed by some disorders, can affect their progress into adult roles.

Socialisation

Peer relationships play an important part in adolescent development and being part of the group. Friends have been identified as a significant factor in the development of social skills and a valuable supportive network during the transition to adulthood (Garrison and McQuiston, 1989; Strax, 1991).

The support of peers during this period is often evaluated negatively, in terms of being at the expense of the parental relationship. Parental relationships are viewed as supportive whereas peer relationships are seen as less supportive and more erratic, providing a negative influence through 'peer pressure' to undertake risk behaviours such as smoking or drinking alcohol, and at times putting obstacles in the way of the chronically ill child in following treatment regimes (Garrison and McQuiston, 1989; Eiser, 1993). However, this may be a simplistic explanation of a complex issue. A study by La Greca (1990) found that the peers of adolescents with diabetes, although considered less supportive than the parents, rather than being obstructive were helpful in making allowances at meal times and in exercise, and provided 'emotional' support for their chronically ill friends. Thus, it may be that parents and peers offer different kinds of support and the chronically ill adolescent may feel more comfortable discussing some issues with friends who have similar 'adolescent' concerns and worries.

Chronic illness has different consequences for social interaction depending on the specifics of the condition and its limitations, and other factors such as age and gender.

La Greca (1990) suggests that diseases which limit physical exercise and daily activities, or alter physical appearance, are likely to have a greater impact on social adjustment. Acceptance of chronically ill children by their peers is often related to the child's observable symptoms and the degree to which they interfere with group participation. Children who 'look different' and cannot join in are an obvious target for ridicule and rejection. The result can be a withdrawal from social situations in order to prevent upset, in turn leading to further isolation from peers and so further reducing the possibility of the development of social skills.

Summary

1   Adolescence is a period of major physiological, psychological and social changes with the main task being to reduce dependence on parents and gain adult independence.

2   The presence of a chronic illness can affect the development of an adolescent's identity by delaying the onset of puberty, by reducing opportunities for social interaction due to illness and by magnifying the feelings of inadequacy and change.

3   Both periods of acute illness and the ongoing treatments for chronic illness can interfere with the adolescent's achievement of independence due to the consequent reliance on parental and medical support.

Conclusion

The impact of chronic illness on a child's development is modified by the essential tasks that need to be achieved at each developmental stage. It is important to assess the factors that may interfere with the development of chronically ill children and to utilise strategies that will minimise the negative impact of chronic illness so enabling chronically ill children to achieve their optimum development potential.

Implications for practice

To enable a child with a chronic illness to achieve their growth and development, potential practitioners need to consider the following:

1 Taking account of how chronic illness may interfere with the attainment of the key developmental tasks at each stage of development throughout childhood.

2 Taking steps to reduce possible childhood misconceptions about chronic illness and treatment in order to minimise hindrances and foster positive adaptation to the chronic illness.

3 Management strategies specific to a child's physical, emotional, intellectual and psychosocial development are needed to ensure that every child is provided with the appropriate opportunities to enhance the achievement of their growth and developmental potential.

References

Anderson BJ (1995) In: Kelnar CJH ed. *Childhood and Adolescent Diabetes.* Chapman Hall, London

Armour S (1991) Andrew. In: Cooper A, Harper V eds. *This is our Child. How Parents Experience The Medical World.* Oxford University Press, Oxford

Barrett H (1991) Jackie. In: Cooper A, Harper V eds. *This is our Child. How Parents Experience The Medical World.* Oxford University Press, Oxford

Baumrind D (1987) A developmental perspective on adolescent risk-taking in contemporary America. In: Irwin CE ed. (1987) *Adolescent Social Behaviour.* Jossey Bass, San Francisco

Bibbace R, Walsh B (1980) Development of children's concepts of illness. *Pediatr* **66**: 912–7

Bowlby J (1969) *Attachment and Loss, Vol 1.* Basic Books, New York

Bradford R (1997) *Children, families and chronic disease: psychological models and methods of care.* Routledge Publications, London

Brietmayer BJ, Gallo AM, Knafl KA *et al* (1992) Social competence of school-aged children with chronic illnesses. *J Pediatr Nurs* **7**(3): 181–7

Cerreto MC (1986) Developmental issues in chronic illness: implications and applications. Topics in Early Childhood Special Education **5**(4): 23–35

Dragone MA (1990) Perspectives of chronically ill adolescents and parents on healthcare needs. *J Pediatr Nurs* **16**(1): 45–9, 108

Eiser C, Town C (1987) Teachers' concerns about chronically ill children. Implications for Pediatricians. *Dev Med Child Neurol* **29**: 53–63

Eiser C (1993) *Growing Up With a Chronic Disease. The Impact on Children and their Families.* Jessica Kingsley Publications, London

Eiser C (1980) How leukaemia affects schooling. *Br J Soc Clin Psychol* **19**: 36–8

Erickson EH (1959) Identity and the life cycle. *Psychol Issues* **1**: 18–164

Erickson EH (1964) *Childhood and Society.* 2nd edn. Norton, New York

Frauman AC, Brandon DH (1996) Toilet training for the child with chronic illness. *J Pediatr Nurs* **22**(6): 469–72

Garrison WT, McQuiston S (1989) *Chronic Illness During Childhood and Adolescence.* Sage Publication, Newbury Park

Gray DE (1993) Perceptions of stigma; parents of autistic children. *Sociol Health Ill* **15**(1): 103–20

Goldberg S, Morris P, Simmons RJ *et al* (1990) Chronic illness in infancy and parenting stress. A comparison of three disease groups. *J Pediatr Psychol* **15**: 347–58

Hauser ST (1991) *Adolescents and their Families: Paths of Ego Development.* Free Press, New York

Irwin CE ed. (1987) *Adolescent Social Behaviour and Health.* Jossey Bass, San Francisco

Kelnar CJH ed. (1995) *Childhood and Adolescent Diabetes.* Chapman Hall, London

La Greca AM (1990) Social consequences of paediatric conditions: A fertile area for future investigation and intervention? *J Pediatr Psychol* **15**: 423–36

Lester B, Zeskind PS (1979) The organisation and assessment of crying in the infant at risk. In: Field T, Sostek A, Goldberg S *et al* eds. (1979) *Infants Born at Risk.* SP Medical and Scientific Books, New York

Linde LM, Rosof B, Dunne OJ *et al* (1966) Attitudinal factors in congenital heart disease. *Pediatr* **38**: 92–101

Manworren RC (1996) Developmental effects on the adolescent of a temporary ileostomy. *J Wound Ostomy Continence Nurs* **23**(4): 210–17

Marcia JE (1982) Identity in adolescence. In: Anderson J ed. *Handbook of adolescent psychology.* John Wiley, Chichester

Neumark-Steiner D, Story M, Resnick D (1995) Body dissatisfaction and unhealthy weight control practices among adolescents with and without chronic illness. A population-based study. *Arch Pediatr Adolesc Med* **1491**: 1330–5

Norton-Fowler MG, Johnson MP, Atkinson SS (1985) School achievement and absence in children with chronic health conditions. *J Pediatr* **106**: 683–7

Park KA, Waters E (1989) Security of attachment and pre-school friendship. *Child Dev* **60**: 1076–81

Patterson JM (1988) Chronic illness and the impact on families. In: Chilman S, Nunally EW, Cox FM eds. *Chronic illness and disability. Families in trouble.* Vol. 2. Sage Publication, Newbury Park

Perrin EC, Gerritty PS (1984) Development of children with chronic illness. *Pediatr* **67**: 841–9

Piaget J (1929) *The Child's Conception of the World.* Harcourt Brace Jovanovich, New York

Piaget J (1952) *The Origins of Intelligence in Children.* International Universities Press, New York

Strax TE (1991) Psychological issues faced by adolescents and young adults with disabilities. *Pediatr Ann* **20**: 507–12

Vessey JA, Swanson MN (1996) Chronic conditions and child development. In: Jackson P (1996) *Primary care of the child with a chronic condition.* 2nd edn. St Louis, Mosby

Wasserman GA, Allen R (1985) Maternal withdrawal from handicapped toddlers. *J Child Psychol Psychiatry* **26**: 381–7

Weitzman M (1984) School and peer relations. *Ped Clin N Am* **31**: 59–69

Wells PW *et al* (1994) Growing up in the Hospital. *J Pediatr Nurs* **9**(2): 66–73

Wright B (1960) *Physical Disability: A psychological approach.* Harper & Bros, New York

Wysoki T, Huxtable D, Linshied T (1989) Adjustment to diabetes mellitus in pre-schoolers and their mothers. *Diabetes Care* **12**: 524–9

Yoos L (1987) Chronic childhood illness: developmental issues. *J Pediatr Nurs* **18**: 25–8

Additional quotes obtained through conversations with families. Names have been changed to protect confidentiality. Used with permission.

4

Children with a chronic illness in pain: strategies for assessment and management of a child in pain

Introduction

'Pain hurts — stupid!' (Carter, 1994). This quotation perhaps best sums up what it is like for a child to be in pain. All children will experience pain at some time in their lives, but children with chronic illness often suffer many kinds of pain as a result of their disorder throughout the whole of their lives. The pain that such a child undergoes may be continual or episodic in nature. It has the capacity to affect every aspect of the child's experience and subsequently affects the family's life.

Children with chronic illness face a lifetime of coping. They have to deal with pain — such as joint pain in rheumatoid arthritis — and discomfort as a result of the ongoing nature of their illness. They have to cope with such procedures as blood tests, bone marrow aspiration, and intravenous drugs. They have to contend with the treatments for their disorder, such as bone marrow transplant or radiotherapy. The effect can be all-consuming as it touches all of the child's experiences and makes 'normal' childhood tasks more difficult to undertake. The presence of ulcers in a child's mouth as a result of chemotherapy means the child will be unwilling to eat or drink because of the discomfort. Or a child will be unwilling to engage in play if moving a limb hurts. Thus, pain interferes with children's ability to cope with everyday life and this, in turn, interferes with their ability to achieve developmental tasks.

Coping with a child suffering from a chronic illness can be stressful for the whole family as the members learn to adapt to meet the ongoing needs of the child and the family unit. This process can become more difficult if the child is in pain. However, it is not just that the child has pain but it is the duration and the context of that pain. As one mother commented:

'It took me a long time to realise that unless she had her therapy she wasn't going to get any better, and even if it hurts

at the time, after she felt a hundred per cent better.'

(Jerrett, 1996)

Yet a child who is in continual pain can be difficult to cope with, as the parents may feel helpless and then focus on finding ways to reduce the pain, often to the exclusion of everything else. As the mother of an eight-year-old child with arthritis noted:

> *'It was hard to do anything at first because if you tried to move her she cried out and I used to try and find ways to make it easier. Now it seems that the pain is easier. She still has a bit when we do the treatment but it's not like it was. She seems so much happier.'*

Nurses and healthcare professionals may not always appreciate the all-consuming effect that pain can have on a child and family. However, in order to help the family to cope with the process of adaptation to chronic illness and to enable the child to achieve his or her optimum growth and development potential, it is essential that pain is controlled. This will improve both the child's and the family's quality of life.

Defining pain

'Pain' has been defined as an unpleasant sensory and emotional experience which is associated with actual or potential tissue damage, or it is described in terms of such damage. It is an individual and subjective phenomenon, and therefore everyone has their own perceptions about pain. 'Pain is whatever the experiencing person says it is, existing whenever he says it does' (McCaffery, 1972). Each individual learns the meaning of the word through experiences related to injury early in life (IASP, 1979). However, it may be difficult for children to define pain as they have limited life experiences and are still developing and so often have difficulty in locating and describing their pain (Carter, 1994). Pain is often defined in terms of its duration as either acute or chronic, but the boundaries between the two are not always clear.

Acute pain

This is usually defined as being of a relatively short duration — less than six months — and diminishes as healing takes place. However, the child experiencing acute pain is unlikely to perceive the experience as brief.

Chronic pain

This is defined as pain that persists beyond the usual course of an acute disease, or which is associated with an underlying chronic condition (IASP, 1979). However, this does not illustrate all aspects of chronic pain and McCaffery and Beebe (1989) further sub-divide chronic or prolonged pain into:

- recurrent acute pain
- ongoing time limited (sometimes referred to as chronic acute pain)
- chronic non-malignant (sometimes referred to as chronic 'benign' pain).

These categories are explained further in *Table 4.1*.

Table 4.1: Types of pain (McCaffery and Beebe, 1989)		
Recurrent acute pain	• can occur over a lifetime • self-contained, predictable episodes • pain free between episodes	eg. sickle-cell pain or migraine
Ongoing time limited pain	• lasts over a prolonged period • high probability will end once cause is cured or controlled	eg. burns pain
Chronic non-malignant pain	• lasts over a long period • emotionally and physically destructive • often non-responsive to available or conventional treatment methods	eg. rheumatoid arthritis pain

Chronic pain in children

Chronic pain for children with a chronic illness is particularly difficult to manage. Indeed, as Carter (1994) states, one of the fundamental differences between acute and chronic pain for children and their families is the impact of the pain upon everyone's lives. Beales (1986) found that for children with juvenile chronic arthritis, chronic pain might be a cause for profound misery. Indeed, chronic pain can disturb the child's emotional, physical and social development (Hodges *et al*, 1985; Webster, 1993). Therefore, chronic pain affects many aspects of a child's life and the lives of other family members, and it has this capacity simply because, by its very nature, it is prolonged.

The child's perception of pain

Pain is a 'complex developmental phenomenon' (Warni, 1990) and this aspect needs to be evaluated carefully when exploring a child's perception of pain. As children develop, their ability to articulate and to understand what is happening regarding their pain management changes. As Carter (1994) suggested, this development parallels their understanding in general. *Table 4.2* on *page 53* (taken from Twycross, 1998a) provides an outline of how children's concepts of pain develop as they mature.

The way in which a child experiences pain is not only modified by a number of developmental issues, but is also modified by various environmental, behavioural and emotional factors. The following are included amongst these factors:

- the characteristics of the child such as age, gender, cognitive level, previous experience, family background
- the coping style of the child
- parental response
- ability of the child to control the situation
- emotional response of the child such as fear, anger or frustration
- the type, duration and intensity of the pain experience.

Table 4.2: How children perceive the cause and effect of pain (Hurley and Whelan, 1988)	
Piaget's stages of development	**Perception of pain**
Preoperational (2–7 years)	• Pain is primarily a physical experience • Think about the magical disappearance of pain • Not able to distinguish between cause and effect of pain • Pain is often perceived as punishment for wrongdoing or bad thoughts (Gildea and Quirk, 1977) particularly if the child did something they were told not to do immediately before they started experiencing pain • Children's egocentricity means that they hold someone else responsible for their pain and therefore are likely to strike out verbally or physically when they experience pain • Child is apt to tell a nurse who gave them an injection, 'You are mean!' (McCaffery, 1972)
Concrete operational (7–11 years)	• Relate to pain physically • Able to specify location in terms of body parts • Increased awareness of the body and internal organs means that fear of bodily harm is a strong influence in their perception of painful events • Fear of total annihilation (body destruction and death) enters their thinking (Schultz, 1971; Alex and Ritchie, 1992)
Transitional formal (10–12 years)	• Have a perception of pain which is not quite as sophisticated as formal-operational children • Their perception of pain is not as literal as would be expected in children who are in the concrete-operational stage of development • Children are beginning to understand the concept of IF... THEN propostitions
Formal operational (12 years and above)	• Begin to solve problems • Do not always have required coping mechanisms to facilitate consistent, mature responses • Imagine the sinister implications of pain (Muller *et al*, 1986)

Parents' perceptions of the child's pain

Ferrell *et al* (Part 1, 1994) asked parents of children with cancer about the impact of pain on the family. The parents felt that often the child's pain was not taken seriously either by the healthcare providers or by other family members when an immediate cause could not be found. Parents also felt that they were fully aware of their child's normal behaviour and were able to discern pain through non-verbal clues despite the child showing no outward behaviours. The parents felt helpless at seeing their child in severe pain. There were expectations from the child that the parents would provide comfort, and the parents had feelings of helplessness and failure when the child's expectations were not met. Parents' identification with the pain was so strong, they stated that they sometimes felt the pain physically. Many parents felt unprepared to deal with relieving pain at home and were quite willing to stay in hospital to avoid having to do so. They felt that the pain experience compounded the already existing nightmare of the cancer diagnosis and described it as horrible/frightening.

Thus, chronic pain associated with chronic illness can be seen to affect the parents as well as the child. Parents of chronically ill children are often able to tell that their child is in pain by the child's non-verbal pain behaviours, and should therefore be encouraged to participate in the management of their child's pain. Healthcare professionals need to involve parents in this aspect of care. If pain is to be taken seriously it is important that healthcare professionals evaluate a child's or a parent's complaint of a child's pain fully, even if an immediate cause cannot be found.

Assessment

In order to help a child with a chronic illness to cope with painful experiences, it is important to assess their pain to be able to provide appropriate management strategies. This can be done in a number of ways and if the child is old enough they should always be involved in assessing their own pain. There are a number of assessment strategies that may be utilised, including:

- pain assessment tools
- pain diaries
- pain history.

Pain assessment tools

There are a number of pain assessment tools available for use with children of different ages. (See Carter, 1994 and Twycross *et al*, 1998b for further information about pain assessment tools). The chronically ill child may have a 'favourite' pain assessment tool, and should be allowed some choice as to which tool is used.

Pain diary

When a child has chronic pain the use of a diary is helpful as it makes it possible to see how the present treatment is working, and to establish when the pain occurs and what is causing the child's pain. Taylor (1988) states that diaries are particularly useful in the assessment of chronic pain. They may include a numerical rating scale and verbal descriptors (McGrath *et al*, 1993), and also enable children to document any episodes of pain and to explore their experience of pain (Carter, 1994). Diaries may, however, result in the child focusing on their pain more than they want to.

Pain history

Liley (1998) suggests that when considering how to treat chronic pain it is important to try to ascertain its cause. A good history is vital and this must be supported by a physical examination and appropriate investigations. When assessing children's pain it is important to consider their stage of cognitive development as children perceive the cause and effect of pain differently at each stage.Using language that may be understood by the child, the nature of the pain should be determined. Remember that children in pain may show signs of regression. Recent analgesic interventions and how well the child is controlling pain should be noted as this might give clues to disease progression or the development of tolerance to drugs which have been used over a long period. The psychological impact of the diagnosis on the patient and the family should be assessed as this may alter the severity of the painful experience. Potential routes to pain relief and the administration of analgesics should be considered.

Management of pain

Melzack and Wall (1982) state that they have learnt, from the results of literally hundreds of experiments, that there is a limit to the effectiveness of any given therapy; but happily the effects of two or more therapies given in conjunction are cumulative. The management of chronic pain in children, therefore, requires the use of both analgesic drugs and appropriate non-drug methods of pain relief.

Analgesic drugs

Analgesics should be tried in a logical sequence based on a ladder of efficacy (WHO, 1990). They should be given by mouth whenever possible (DTB, 1995a) and should be given regularly and in adequate doses. Paracetamol, non-steroid anti-inflammatory drugs (NSAID's), codeine and morphine together with local anaesthetics should meet most needs (DTB, 1995b), although it must be remembered that a combination of opioid and non-opioid drugs is often more effective given together rather than separately.

Many of the stronger analgesic drugs have side effects, such as drowsiness and nausea, that may affect the child's quality of life. It is important when devising a plan of care to manage chronic pain that the child and their family are involved in the decision-making process. They will be able to decide when either the pain intensity or the side effects become intolerable. In some cases there needs to be a balance between the child's functional ability and a reduction in the pain experience (Carter, 1994; Newburger and Sallan, 1981). There is a need to find a balance between the child's quality of life and an acceptable level of side effects from the analgesic drugs. Only the child and his or her family can decide what is acceptable.

The child with a chronic illness may be taking other drugs, so when deciding on a pain management plan it is important to consider the interaction between different drugs in order to minimise side effects. When considering a treatment strategy Liley (1998) suggests that the aim should be to manage the pain adequately while avoiding, as far as possible, significant side effects. This balance is different for each child and any regime must be tailored to fit the individual's needs. Liley (1998) also suggests that the problems associated with taking certain analgesics need to be anticipated and addressed at an early stage; for example, laxatives should be given to a child on strong opiates. Discussion with the family and the child should take place to dispel any fears and misconceptions that they may have, particularly if the child requires strong opiates as there is a general — if largely overplayed — fear of dependence and addiction. Liley (1998) states that good pain control is dependent on the use of appropriate agents:

- at an appropriate dosage
- via an appropriate route
- at appropriate frequencies.

The management of chronic pain often requires the use of adjuvant drugs. It is important to remember that adjuvant drugs are not a substitute for adequate doses of opioids and non-opioid analgesics. Aggressive titration of analgesics to control pain comes first. Then, if additional symptoms remain, adjuvant drugs can be added (McCaffery and Beebe, 1994). Types of adjuvant drugs include some antidepressants, some anti-convulsants, some muscle relaxants and occasionally steroids. Further information about adjuvant drugs can be found in McCaffery and Beebe (1994).

Non-drug methods

Non-drug methods of pain control are probably most effective as coping strategies, and not for actual reduction of the intensity of pain. Although there are exceptions to this statement, such as the use of cold, the most likely outcome of techniques such as relaxation and distraction is that the pain will be more tolerable, not necessarily less severe in intensity (McCaffery and Wong, 1993). Many non-drug techniques can be taught or facilitated by nurses so that the child and their family can take over this part of their pain management (Carter, 1994). This allows them some control over the management of the pain. Non-drug methods of pain control may be overused or even abused with certain children or in selected circumstances. Children who are co-operative and adept at techniques such as distraction may actually suffer in silence and not be provided with appropriate analgesia or local anesthesia (McCaffery and Wong 1993). Adequate analgesic drugs must be used as and when necessary; additional methods of reducing pain and anxiety will help the child to relax and cope better with pain and distress (May 1992).

Sometimes non-drug methods alone will be adequate. Generally, however, they are used in conjunction with drug and other non-drug methods. Not all patients will find them beneficial (Twycross 1994).

Table 4.3 on *pages 60–61* provides a summary of some of the more common non-drug methods available for the relief of pain.

It is important to remember that children who are using distraction techniques and other non-drug methods of pain relief may not look as if they are in pain. Nurses and other healthcare professionals need to remember that non-drug methods do not take away the pain; they dull the child's perception of the pain. Non-drug methods should, therefore, be used in conjunction with analgesic drugs.

Twycross (1998c) states that healthcare professionals and parents can use many of the non-drug methods described in this chapter with very little training. Other non-drug methods, such as aromatherapy and hypnosis, require a recognised qualification to be obtained. It is important that healthcare professionals do not implement methods of which they have little or no knowledge. Utilising the skills of the multi-disciplinary team is important; play therapists and clinical psychologists have a vital role in implementing non-drug methods.

Procedural pain

Children with chronic illness often endure many painful procedures. Fear and anxiety about painful processes often increases when the procedure is repeated and may intensify the pain experienced by the child (Jay *et al*, 1983). Psychological and contextual factors need to be considered. McGrath (1986) points out that a lumbar puncture may elicit different pain responses in different children. A child with cancer, who has just relapsed, may perceive more pain than a child who is in remission and completing treatment. McGrath (1986) found that the following helped a child to cope with lumbar punctures:

- deep breathing, relaxation exercises
- visual imagery
- a parent's or nurse's hand on the child's shoulder
- encouraging the child to squeeze someone's finger during the lumbar puncture to correspond to the amount of pain they feel
- teaching the child to concentrate on making their back numb, or moving pain from their back, along their arm and out through their hand
- talking to the child to help 'take their mind off' the pain.

These methods could also be utilised to help children cope with other painful procedures. The involvement of play therapists and clinical psychologists, when appropriate, at an early stage will ensure that children are prepared for painful procedures.

Summary

1 A child with chronic illness often suffers pain. This pain may be continual, episodic or due to the painful effects of the disease, procedures and/or treatments, and has the capacity to affect all areas of the child's life and that of their family.

2 The aim of care is to reduce the impact of pain and to balance the effects of relieving the pain with the unacceptable side effects of some of the stronger analgesics.

Implications for practice

In order to reduce the impact of pain on a child with a chronic illness, the nurse and health professional need to do the following.

1 Ensure that before planing a child's pain management his or her pain needs are assessed using a pain assessment tool.

2 Utilise management strategies which make use of both analgesic drugs and non-drug methods to control pain. Some non-drug methods can be particularly useful in helping children to cope with procedural pain.

Table 4.3: Non-drug methods of pain relief (Twycross, 1998b)

Distraction	• Best with relatively short duration pain such as procedural pain (Carter, 1994) • Makes pain more tolerable or bearable by putting pain at the periphery of awareness (McCaffery and Beebe, 1989) • Attention is focused on the distracter rather than the pain (Carter, 1994) • To determine an effective distraction strategy the nurse involves the child and parents in identifying what is particularly interesting to the child (McCaffery and Wong, 1993)
Relaxation	• Does not reduce the intensity of pain but reduces the distress associated with pain (Carter, 1994) • A patient cannot be relaxed and anxious concurrently; pain tolerance should be increased if the patient is relaxed (Weisenberg, 1980) • An effective coping strategy for procedural, chronic or ongoing pain (McCaffery and Wong, 1993) • For pain that lasts most of the day a relaxation technique may be performed several times a day (McCaffery and Wong, 1993) • Ideally taught prior to painful procedures
Touch	• A two-way process involving sensation and cognition (Carter, 1994) • The need to be touched is present at birth and is a continuing and developing need (Carter, 1995) • Provides one of the strongest means of communicating caring and empathy (Carter, 1994)
Transcutaneous electric nerve stimulation (TENS)	• Useful in localised pain — thought to increase endorphin levels and act as a counter irritant (McCaffery and Beebe, 1989) • Little research in its use in paediatrics (Eland, 1993) • Should be used in combination with other treatment methods (Eland, 1993) • TENS aims to relieve pain and is non-invasive and safe (Eland, 1993) • the TENS device delivers controlled low voltage electricity to the body via electrodes (Eland, 1993) • TENS recipients often describe a sensation of tingling when the device is working (McCaffery and Beebe, 1989) • Useful for both acute and chronic pain (Sofaer, 1992)

Imagery	• The use of imagination to modify the response to pain (Doody *et al*, 1991) • Involves using sensory images which modify the pain to make it more bearable or substitute a pleasant image in place of pain (McCaffery and Beebe, 1989) • Can be used in a guided way so that the child imagines something about their pain flowing out of their body (Carter, 1994)
Massage	• The systematic manual manipulation of the soft tissues of the body to produce relaxation of the muscles (Beck, 1988) • Promotes circulation of the blood, relief from pain, restoration of metabolic balance as well as other physical and emotional benefits (Beck, 1988) • An ancient method of maintaining and improving health (McCaffery and Beebe, 1989)
Aromatherapy	• An holistic form of healing which uses essential oils extracted from aromatic plants (Carter, 1995) • Increasingly used as a means of reducing stress, relaxing, treating symptoms and providing relief from pain (Carter, 1995) • Promotes healing on different levels — physical, emotional and mental (Carter, 1995) • Should only be practised by a trained practitioner (Carter, 1995)
Acupuncture	• A system of ancient medicine, healing and Eastern philosophy originating in China (Yee *et al*, 1993) • The Chinese explanation of how acupuncture works is based on the idea that life force flows round certain lines on the body known as meridians (Mayer *et al*, 1976) • Needling points on these lines is thought to correct an abnormal flow of life force (Mann, 1971) • Another explanation is that acupuncture stimulates the production of natural endorphins (Mayer *et al*, 1976) • Particularly helpful in treating chronic pain; not effective in treating advanced cancer pain (Sofaer, 1992)
Hypnosis	• Defined as focused attention, an altered state of consciousness or a trance, often accompanied by relaxation (Valente, 1991) • Found to be of value in the care and management of children with both acute and chronic pain (Carter, 1994) • Does not actually take away the pain but decreases/removes the child's perception of it (Carter, 1994)

References

Alex JA, Ritchie MR (1992) School-aged children's interpretation of their experience with acute surgical pain. *J Pediatr Nurs* **7**(3): 171–80

Beales G (1986) Cognitive development and the experience of pain. *Nursing* **11**: 408–410

Beck M (1988) *The Theory and Practice of Therapeutic Massage.* Milady, New York

Carter B (1994) *Child and Infant Pain: Principles of Nursing Care and Management.* Chapman and Hall, London

Carter B (1995) Complementary therapies and the management of chronic pain. *Paediatr Nurs* **7**(3):18–22

Doody SB, Smith C, Webb J (1991) Non-pharmacological interventions for pain management. *Critical Care Nurs Clin North Am* **3**(1): 69–75

DTB (1995a) Managing pain in children. *DTB* **33**: 41–4

DTB (1995b) Managing chronic pain in children. *DTB* **33**(7): 52–5

Eland J (1993) The Use of TENS with Children. In: Schechter NL, Berde CB, Yaster M eds. *Pain in Infants, Children and Adolescents.* Williams and Wilkins, Baltimore

Ferrell BR, Rhiner M, Shapiro B *et al* (1994) The experience of pediatric cancer pain, part 1: Impact of pain on the family. *J Pediatr Nurs* **9**(6): 368–79

Ferrell BR, Rhiner M, Shapiro B *et al* (1994) The experience of pediatric cancer pain, part 2: Management of pain. *J Pediatr Nurs* **9**(6): 380–7

Gildea JH, Quirk JH, Quirk TH (1977) Assessing the pain experience in children. *Nurs Clin North Am* No.1

Hodges K, Kline JJ, Barbero G *et al* (1985) Depressive symptoms in children with recurrent abdominal pain and their families. *J Pediatr* **107**: 622–6

Hurley A, Whelan EG (1988) Cognitive development and children's perception of pain. *Pediatr Nurs* **14**(1): 21–4

International Association of the Study of Pain, Subcommittee on Taxonomy (1979) Pain terms: A list with definitions and notes on usage. *Pain* **6**: 249–52

Jay SM *et al* (1983) Assessment of children's distress during painful procedures. *Health Psychol* **2**:133–47

Jerrett MD (1996) Parents' experiences of coming to know the care of a chronically ill child. In: Smith JP (1996) *Nursing Care of Children. Advanced Nursing Series.* Blackwell Scientific Publications, Oxford

Liley A (1998) The management of chronic pain. In: Twycross A, Moriarty A, Betts T eds. *Paediatric Pain Management: A Multi-disciplinary Approach.* Radcliffe Medical Press, Oxford

Mann F (1971) Chapter 3 In: Sofaer B (1992) *Pain: A Handbook for Nurses.* 2nd edn. Chapman and Hall, London

May L (1992) Reducing pain and anxiety in children. *Nurs Stand* **6**(4): 25–8

Mayer DJ, Price DD, Raffii A (1976) Antagonism and acupuncture analgesia in man by the narcotic antagonist naloxone. *Brain Res* 368–77

McCaffery M (1972) *Nursing Management of the Patient with Pain.* Lippincott, Philadelphia

McCaffery M, Beebe AB (1989) *Pain: Clinical Manual for Nursing Practice.* C V Mosby, St Louis

McCaffery M, Beebe AB (1994) *Pain: Clinical Manual for Nursing Practice.* UK edn. C V Mosby, London

McCaffery M, Wong D (1993) Nursing interventions for pain control in children. In: Schechter NL, Berde CB, Yaster M eds. *Pain in Infants, Children and Adolescents.* Williams and Wilkins, Baltimore

McGrath PA (1986) Helping children with painful procedures. *AJN* November: 1278–9

McGrath PJ, Ritchie JA, Unrah AM (1993) Paediatric Pain. In: Carroll D, Bowsher D eds. *Pain Management and Nursing Care.* Butterworth-Heinemann,Oxford

Melzack R, Wall PD (1982) *The Challenge of Pain.* Penguin Books, London

Muller DJ, Harris PJ, Wattley L (1986) *Nursing Children: Psychology, Research and Practice.* Harper and Rowe, London

Newburger PE, Sallan SE (1981) Chronic pain: principles of management. *J Pediatr* **98**:180–9

Schultz NV (1971) How children perceive pain. *Nurs Outlook* 670–3

Sofaer B (1992) Pain: A Handbook for Nurses. 2nd edn. Chapman and Hall, London

Taylor A (1998) Pain assessment in children. In: Twycross A, Moriarty A, Betts T eds. (1998) *Paediatric Pain Management: A Multi-disciplinary Approach.* Radcliffe Medical Press, Oxford

Twycross A, Moriarty A, Betts T eds. (1998) *Paediatric Pain Management: A Multi-Disciplinary Approach.* Radcliffe Medical Press, Oxford

Twycross A (1998a) Children's cognitive level and their perceptions of pain. In: Twycross A, Moriarty A, Betts T eds. *Paediatric Pain Management: A Multi-disciplinary Approach.* Radcliffe Medical Press, Oxford

Twycross A (1998b) The assessment and management of pain in children. *Prof Nurse* **14**(2): 95–8

Twycross A (1998c) Non-drug methods of pain control. In: Twycross A, Moriarty A, Betts T eds. *Paediatric Pain Management: A Multi-disciplinary Approach.* Radcliffe Medical Press, Oxford

Twycross RG (1994) *Pain Relief in Advanced Cancer.* Churchill Livingstone, London

Valente SM (1991) Using hypnosis with children for pain management. *Oncol Nurs Forum* **18**(4):699–704

Warni JW (1990) Behavioural management of pain in children. In Tyler DC, Krane EJ eds. *Advances in Research Therapy Volume 15* Raven Press, New York

Webster DE (1993) Chronic and recurrent pain during childhood. In: Ramamurthy S, Roger JN eds. *Decision-Making in Pain Management.* Mosby, St Louis

Weisenberg M (1980) Understanding pain phenomena. In: Carter B (1994) *Child and Infant Pain: Principles of Nursing Care and Management.* Chapman and Hall, London

WHO (1990) *Cancer Pain Relief and Palliative Care (Tech Rep Ser 804).* WHO, Geneva

Yee JD, Lin YC, Aubuchon PA (1993) Acupuncture. In: Schechter NL, Berde CB, Yaster M eds. *Pain in Infants, Children and Adolescents.* Williams and Wilkins, Baltimore

Additional quotes obtained through conversations with families. Names have been changed to protect confidentiality. Used with permission.

5

Chronic illness and the family: the effects on family interaction

Introduction

Parenting a sick child is a normal family experience. All children become ill and have periods of acute illness, or accidents which may require medical intervention or hospital admission. Parents have to find a way of dealing with their emotions while meeting the needs of the sick child and the family. However, parenting a child with a chronic illness is different; the long-term nature means that 'what was originally called an emergency can become an everyday part of life' (Altschuler, 1997). The diagnosis of chronic illness places 'special' demands on the family, disrupting 'normal family life' and requiring substantive changes in the family structure, function and role responsibilities as members learn to adapt to the new care demands (Hauerstein, 1990).

Understanding a parent's perspective

For a health professional, there is a tendency to describe chronic illness or disability in objective terms and not to appreciate the profound impact a diagnosis can have on the family. As Hilary Freeman (1991) explained when talking of her daughter, Julia:

> 'So here we are with a child who is in medical and educational language profoundly handicapped. She can do nothing for herself and has just about no controlled movement at all... However, such an objective description says nothing about Julia herself and it is not the way we see her day-to-day.'
>
> (Freeman, 1991)

For the family, chronic illness has far-reaching practical and emotional consequences. Family members have to adjust to the news that the disease and treatment is for life, affecting relationships, everyday routines and the aspirations parents have for their children (Eiser, 1993; Bradford, 1997).

The family

Most of us have experienced a family and that experience leaves us with strongly held beliefs about what a family is and how a family should care for its members. However, defining what constitutes a family can create a number of difficulties. Although research of families has tended to focus on the traditional model of a nuclear family with mother, father and siblings and how they have adapted to chronic illness, this may not be the makeup of all families (Bradford, 1997).

The narrow focus on traditional models of family makeup can result in obscuring such variations in family composition as single parents, same-sex relationships and the impact and important wider family support provided by others such as grandparents.

Defining the family

Whall (1986) analysed the concept of the family as a self-identified group of two or more people whose association is defined by special terms and who function as a family. A family is acknowledged as being the 'basic unit of society' (Keller, 1977; Terkelson, 1980) which exists to nurture the members of the family group. Although the composition of each family group can vary, the central purpose of the family is to create and maintain a common culture which promotes the growth and well-being of and provides physical and emotional support for each of its members (Terkelson, 1980). This indicates that family life is crucial to human and social development (Whyte, 1994). While it may be argued that this function could be achieved by any social group, families differ in a number of ways that include the following:

- relationships or bonds are primarily affectionate. Although affection can grow in relationships other than in families, this is secondary to the common interest that brought the individuals together, such as a religious belief, a job or a hobby
- a family contains a variety of ages and genders with no common interest except being part of the family

- membership is virtually permanent and even after death members become part of family history and culture
- there is social acceptance that family ties are the most important and obligations to the family are often considered more important than any other responsibility.

These attributes place an emphasis on affection, loyalty and durability as essential characteristics of family life and allow the inclusion of the various forms of family groups prevalent in modern society (Wright and Leahey, 1990).

Family members are interdependent with all members affecting one another, so that anything which affects one member will affect the family as a whole (Marshack and Seligman, 1993). Given this reciprocal relationship, a child with chronic illness can have an impact on the whole family functioning. As Burr (1985) stated: 'A dynamic relationship exists between family functioning and the functioning of family members.'

Effects of chronic illness on the family

Each family has its own values, beliefs and structures that define both how family members interact with each other and how the family interacts with the outside world. Family members adapt and alter their ways of working and relating to one another in response to a demand for change. Faced with a chronically ill child member, it is the family who acts as a buffer to absorb the stress and strain of coping with the additional care demands imposed by the illness (Clawson, 1996). The effects of the illness mean the family has to adapt to considerable change in roles, structures and patterns of relating (Altschuler, 1997).

Family responses to chronic illness

The response of the family to caring for a child with chronic illness is determined by the following:

- beliefs within the family organisation
- physical and emotional energy
- intellect
- confidence
- threshold for stress

- the styles adopted when challenged: be this assertive, passive, or optimistic (Walker, 1991).

However, the strategies and ability to cope with chronic illness do not occur in a vacuum. As Altschuler (1997) noted:

> *'While beliefs construct our experience of illness, so too experiences over time construct what we believe.'*

Thus, the ways in which parents and family deal with the impact of chronic illness are affected by past and present experiences of illness and coping with illness. In as much as the parents affect the child, so the child's response to chronic illness affects the parents. This can be seen in the following description by a mother of a 14-year-old boy who was receiving treatment for cancer:

> *'Rory was so good about everything. Even when all his hair fell out he didn't want to wear a hat, even those baseball caps all the others had. He used to spike the few strands that were left with gel into some sort of spikey style!! It wasn't easy and I was proud of how he coped. Some of the other parents didn't have it so easy. It's difficult not to notice when you're all together in hospital...'*

Summary

Each family has its own values, beliefs and structure. The experiences and coping styles of the parents, the chronically ill child and other family members can determine the capacity of the family and the child to deal with problems and adapt to the stresses and changes resulting from chronic illness.

Impact of chronic illness on the family

All families experience stress at one time or another, but families with children who are chronically ill must meet the demands imposed by the illness. Caring for a child with a chronic illness makes a significant impact on the level of practical and emotional stresses for the whole family (Eiser, 1993). Changes to family life as a result of chronic illness can include:

- alterations in family relationships and roles
- limitations on family activities
- limitations on parents' aspirations and goals, both for the child and for themselves, as caring for a sick child may limit personal career aspirations
- increased child-caring tasks
- increased financial burdens
- housing adaptation
- social isolation
- medical concerns about the child's illness and the ability of the medical profession to treat the child
- school experiences including coping with treatments, disability and interruptions due to illness
- the emotional demands of everyday care and the grieving and loss of the healthy, 'perfect' child.

Stress of chronic illness

The stress of chronic illness on family functioning has been recognised since the early 1970s, although the impact of the stress on family functioning is not well understood. Early studies focused on the negative and dysfunctional aspects of family functioning due to profound disruption requiring substantive changes in family structure (Hauerstein, 1990). However, positive effects of a family adapting to chronic illness have also been identified. Miller and Wood (1991) found that successful adaptation by the family can facilitate the healthy growth and development of the chronically ill child. There is also an opportunity for families to 'grow' as a result of their mastery of the chronic illness experiences (Clawson, 1996).

Walker *et al* (1987) compared stress and adjustment in mothers of children who had cystic fibrosis and mothers with 'healthy' children, and found no significant differences in the perceived stress and/or adequacy as parents between the two groups, although mothers of the 'healthy' children reported more child-related problems. Although it appeared that both groups were not significantly dissimilar, it was surprising to note that the families with chronic illness did not always report more problems. However, the findings must be interpreted with care, as families with chronically ill children may not want to acknowledge the difficulties and may have different perceptions of stress and coping within family life. But the study does highlight the dangers both of negatively stereotyping families with chronic illness as having more problems and of labelling such families as dysfunctional. This does not mean that the additional stresses or problems resulting from the illness should be discounted, but rather that families need to be assessed individually in order to determine the impact of the child's illness on daily living.

Family response to chronic illness

How a families deal with the impact of the diagnosis of chronic illness varies. Kazack and Nachman (1991) suggest that the coping strategies of the family before the diagnosis of chronic illness may be critical, influencing the way in which the family reorganises to meet the needs of the ill child. As Gill describes, talking about her eight-year-old son:

> *'Always having Duncan as a semi-sickly child, we've just sort of taken CF in our stride and just keep going... CF has become part of our life and we've put it there, and just carried on the best we could.'*

(Whyte, 1994)

Some families do not cope with the additional demands, and there is evidence to suggest that children from homes with parental conflict are more likely to show emotional and behavioural problems (Block *et al*, 1981). However, many families find they have inner resources of which they were previously unaware, and studies highlight the powerful role parents play in mediating the effects of an illness on a child (Greenburg and Meadows, 1991).

Although not all families consist of the traditional mother, father and siblings, this family structure has been the focus of most of the empirical research. A major concern has been that the focus on the chronically ill child and on the parental role in relation to that child may be at the expense of the marital relationship and other family members. It is the way in which a family, and particularly the parents, perceives and shares the burden of care that seems to be a significant factor in the family's ability to cope with the demands placed on it (Gibson, 1988).

Burden of care

The demands of care for children with a chronic illness can be considerable. For example, for a child with cystic fibrosis the demands of up to an hour of physiotherapy four times daily and the supervision of enzyme replacement along with the monitoring of appetite, stools and weight gain require constant effort and have to be managed within the context of the needs of other family members in order to maintain some sort of 'normal' family life. As the mother of a hearing-impaired child noted:

> *'It's very easy to live your life around the handicapped child, whereas everybody in the family has their own personality that has to be developed and their own interests. So it has to be balanced.'*

(Hornby, 1994)

Added to the stresses of coping with the demands of chronic illness are such normal stresses of life as bereavements, financial worries, academic achievement at school, and so on. With everything taken into account, the cumulative effect can result in minor events taking on the greater significance of 'crisis proportions' (Whyte, 1992). Thus, the help and support of all family members are essential in sharing the burden of care and keeping family life as normal as possible (Whyte, 1994).

Distribution of care

Much of the literature and research has focused on the mothers of chronically ill children, assuming that they have the largest burden of care. This may be true for traditional families, as it is the mother who often manages care (Anderson and Elfert, 1989) and who has the closest contact with the hospital (Eiser, 1993). This greater responsibility for care taken by mothers may mirror the functioning of most families with healthy children (La Rossa, 1986). However, this focus can tend to obscure the issues for other carers in the family and those who do not fit the 'traditional' family makeup. There is little evaluation of single parent families in which the lone parent often has to cope with the stress of the chronically ill child without the support of a partner or wider social networks.

Some research has taken the amount of time parents spent with children, particularly the sick child, as an indicator of the burden of care. However, this may not accurately reflect the distribution of work or care within families and may be an inadequate indicator of parental or carer involvement. The father's involvement with the sick child in a traditional family can be overlooked as he may be the wage-earner and not have the same time to care or be involved in other household duties and managing the needs of other siblings (Cook, 1984). In addition, siblings and grandparents may manage other aspects of different family needs, such as cooking or cleaning, which are not taken into account and yet contribute to the care of the sick child.

Summary

The presence of a chronically ill child in the family has a significant impact on the practical and emotional demands on the family. The effect on family functioning of the stress arising from the chronic illness is influenced by the family dynamics, support, and placing of the burden of care within the family.

Family relationships

Parental relationship: roles and responsibilities

The role of caring for the sick child can create a number of stresses for the parents. Jane was asked how the care of her son, David, aged four, with cystic fibrosis was managed:

> *'I'm the one who gives him his drugs, does the physiotherapy and takes him to clinic. Mark can't; he's working. He does what he can. I wish he could do more. I don't think he realises what I've got to do sometimes... it can be tiring and I get fed up sometimes, but you can't stop... just sometimes it would be good to have a day off... .'*

This quote reflects a traditional view of the distribution of care. It may not be a reflection of all families, but research has highlighted gender differences and coping styles utilised by parents which can affect the perceptions of roles, parenting styles and the quality of the parental relationship.

Role expectations

Cook (1984), studying changing role expectations, found a trend for mothers to assume primary care-taking responsibilities while fathers assumed increased care for other siblings and functioned stoically as breadwinners. This resulted in different experiences for the parents and different attendant concerns. For mothers, increased social isolation, intense involvement with the sick child and medical staff, and a focus on shielding others coloured their experiences. For fathers, the crucial issues were the competing obligations of work and family, and a feeling of being 'left out' of the medical decisions concerning care. Thus, wives feared increasing emotional distance from their husbands, while husbands reported feeling alienated from the sick child and their wives over involvement with the child. These differences in concerns and roles in care can be a source of conflict and stress for parents.

Coping with changing roles is further complicated by the need to evaluate beliefs and practices about child rearing, including discipline and education.

Discipline practices

'Getting it right' and providing a consistent and appropriate parental style of management of a child's day-to-day needs is a constant source of concern for all parents. Parents worry about child rearing; when to restrict behaviour and when to be flexible in managing a child's behaviour. Such worries are particularly problematic when children go through periods of acute illness and require ongoing treatments. The demands of a child with a chronic disease may mean that different parenting practices are required at different times, for example a relaxation of discipline practices when they are ill, which in turn can send mixed messages to the child. Parental dilemmas about child rearing may be further aggravated by the ambiguous nature of chronic illness. As Eiser (1993) noted:

> *'Although the conditions are not curable, many children look normal and do not seem so very different from before diagnosis.'*

Parents' initial concerns following diagnosis of chronic illness focus on the practical requirements of managing the condition on a day-to-day basis. At this time the child may seem very ill and the parents may try to make the child feel special. In responding to the child's pain or discomfort, parents may buy gifts and 'turn a blind eye' to unacceptable behaviours in order to encourage the child to get well. Problems can then occur when these behaviours continue beyond the initial crisis and parents have difficulty in adopting an appropriate parenting style.

The diagnosis of a chronic illness can challenge the parents' current management style in caring for the child. Important parental perceptions include:

- the prognosis of the disorder
- the limitations imposed by the disorder and its treatment
- the child's response to the illness.

These perceptions can affect the decisions the parents have made and will make about parenting, and the way in which they attempt to deal with the restrictions of care on a day-to-day basis.

Parenting management styles

Prior to the diagnosis, the parents may have negotiated clear boundaries for each partner's role and how discipline should be managed. These perceptions and roles may need to be renegotiated as a result of the child's chronic illness.

Treatment programmes can regulate and restrict relationships between the parents and other family members (Eiser, 1993). The parents have to be watchful of a child's needs, such as dietary intake and medication in diabetes. This may not only involve the learning of new tasks but also can force parents to rethink beliefs about personal parental roles, communication and responsibilities of care. All of these issues influence the way the parents manage the care of the family and how they relate to one another, and can create a source of conflict.

According to early research, the parents' response was to adopt an overprotective and restrictive parenting style. The interaction between child and parent was evaluated in terms of excesses of parental behaviour such as overindulgence, increased anxiety, strictness and perfectionism. However, as Eiser (1993) noted, this approach is too narrow, and many of the studies had been based on mothers' reports with little verification through observation. In addition, there are no cohesive theoretical frameworks on parenting, in either families with or without a child with a chronic illness.

The theoretical approaches to parenting have focused on factors that could affect the child-parent relationship. Parenting behaviour may be affected by the:

- emotional state of the parents
- parents' beliefs about parenting
- parents' previous parenting experience (siblings)
- parents' values (balancing personal goals, career aspirations, family life)
- prognosis and course of the chronic illness
- child's reaction to diagnosis
- family's financial stability.

A literature review revealed few studies that have addressed how the family unit responds to chronic illness (Knafl and Deatrick, 1990). Davis (1963), in a classic study of polio victims, described two responses of normalisation and disassociation. This theme has been developed by other researchers who have explored normalisation as a healthy response to chronic illness (Knafl and Daetrick, 1990). However, this glosses over the individual responses of families and the various stages they may go through in adapting to chronic illness.

Knafl *et al* (1996) described a number of management styles in families with chronic illnesses. Although the study is qualitative and therefore the sample is small, it does provide a picture of the diversity of coping styles — on an adaptive to maladaptive continuum of parenting management styles — of families with a chronically ill child (see *Figure 5.1*).

Figure 5.1: Family management styles (Knafl *et al*, 1996)				
Adaptive	→	→	→	*Maladaptive*
Thriving	Accommodating	Enduring	Struggling	Floundering

Thriving The parents and child viewed themselves as 'normal', had an accommodating and proactive management style and made care a part of family life.

Accommodating The parents perceived themselves as responding to the situation and although they coped well with it, they found difficulties accepting the seriousness and possible future complications of the illness.

Enduring The parents held a negative view of the illness and tremendous energy was put into illness management. They emphasised the need to protect the child.

Struggling There was parental conflict about how to manage the child which was grounded on differing views of the illness, expectations of one another's role and participation in care.

Floundering The parents had a negative view of the child's illness and how best to manage it, and there was also evidence of ineffective management.

The experience of chronic illness presents families with multiple challenges and they respond in different ways. However, Knafl *et al* (1996) noted that families who have a philosophy of normality, a similar perception of the disease and management, and share the burden of care, appear to adapt more easily and manage the child's care more effectively. It was noted that families' management styles were not static but changed over time and the progression was not linear. Families may work through a number of styles although the reasons for changes are not always clear. However, where families resolve difficulties and adopt a thriving or accommodating style of management, the child adapts more positively and care is more effectively delivered.

Career aspirations

The diagnosis of chronic illness may also require a change in the roles and relationships in parenting. An example may be where the father loses his job and takes on the caring role which was previously the wife's responsibility, or where the mother gives up career aspirations to become a full-time carer. The diagnosis of illness or disability creates a change in the family perceptions, and possibly aspirations. As a father commented about his experience with Sally, a five year old with Down's syndrome:

> *'Since we had Sally, my wife wanted to be very close to her mother because she gets a lot of support from her. This has meant I was restricted in applying for jobs in the same city where we live, where she could have contact with her mother. We've had constant conflict about me always wanting to move to get promotion. I also had an urge to see the country through teaching as well. This is my personal*

aim if you like, but of course having Sally virtually immobilised us in this area.'

(Hornby, 1994)

The extent to which this factor creates a source of conflict largely depends on the extent and attitude of the family to the changes.

Summary

Caring for a child with a chronic disorder can be a source of stress affecting the parental relationship as roles and responsibilities of care, discipline and future aspirations are evaluated and renegotiated. Families may adopt a number of management styles which can be a help or a hindrance to the child's adaptation to the chronic illness.

Parental (partner) relationship

The changes that occur in the parental (partner) relationship can have a negative impact on family functioning and it has been suggested that this population has a higher incidence of divorce.

Divorce statistics

A comprehensive review of 34 studies by Sabbath and Leventhal (1984) did not support the assumption of a higher incidence of divorce. Few families cite a child's condition as a cause of divorce (Hare *et al*, 1966) but this may not be a good indicator of reasons for divorce as parents may not wish to be seen as blaming the child. However, existing problems in relationships may be magnified by the difficulties of having a child with a chronic illness. As Sabbath and Leventhal (1984) found in a study of families with a child with cancer, the presence of the ill child in the family puts considerable strain on parental relationships, with 33 per cent of parents having depression and anxiety and needing professional help.

These statistics are perhaps not surprising when one considers the stress a chronic illness can create for a family. Alison explains how the diagnosis of her son, six-year-old Pau,l with cancer affected her and consequently the family:

> *'It was hard to cope with all the drugs, and the hospital appointments. I shut myself off from everything else to try and get through it all. Alex was great... he tried to help... I don't know how he put up with me. I used to get irritable and shout at him and Sarah. Sometimes it seemed like that's all we did... argue. I suppose I took it out on him* [silent pause]*... looking back... but, you just try to keep going.'*

This illustrates the impact that the illness can have on all members of the family, and the emotional and physical toll it can have on them as the focus becomes the sick child. The impact on the parental relationship can be profound not only in terms of the parenting role but also of the partner relationship.

Partner relationship

Having and focusing on a child with a chronic illness can cause a negative impact on the relationship between partners due to:

- problems of the illness including ongoing treatment and periods of acute exacerbation of the disease leading to emotional and financial strain
- disruption of social life and social isolation. Families with larger social support networks reported less stress and a greater degree of adjustment to the chronic illness and disability
- the burdens of ongoing family needs in addition to the demands of the chronically ill child.

All of these issues can leave parents with little time or energy for other activities or interpersonal relationships. Even where families remain intact, the quality of the parents' relationship can suffer, with parents of chronically ill children reporting distress and dissatisfaction with their marriage (Donnelly *et al*, 1987). Much of the dissatisfaction appears to stem from a perceived inadequacy of communication between the parents, particularly when there is conflict regarding the sharing of the practical and emotional burdens of child care.

Partner stress

Gill said that if Duncan, eight years old, had a medical problem she would:

'... "see to it" when she was at the clinic or go and see her
GP. "Other than that I just shout and scream at Hugh" (her
husband).'

(Whyte, 1994)

It seems that tensions can be taken out on a partner particularly where
the burden of care is not equally shared. Often the mother bears the
burden of care, and Barbarin *et al* (1985) found that mothers often felt
alone in caring for their child, finding little time for themselves or their
husbands after the demands of child care had been met.

Tension about the burden and perceptions of parental roles can create
dissatisfaction affecting the quality of the relationship between parents.
Lansky *et al* (1978) found more marital distress in families with a child
with cancer than in parents of haemophiliacs or a 'normal' population,
but less stress in couples who were in marital counselling. The marital
stress did not appear to be related to length of time since diagnosis or
death of the child, but seemed to reflect feelings of low self-esteem,
helplessness and strong, unmet dependency needs. The issue of meeting
the needs of the carers is an important one, as the assumption is that the
couple may offer each other support which may enable the family and
child to cope with the effects of the chronic illness.

Meeting partner needs

The importance of ensuring the needs of the carers are met is reflected
in a study by Barbarin *et al* (1985). Although there was little reported
marital stress in families of children with cancer, as the number of
hospitalisations increased perceived marital quality decreased. Thus, as
the burden of care increased the perceived marital quality decreased.
However, there was a difference in what was perceived to be important
regarding the quality of relationships. Wives perceived a connection
between the quality of their relationship and their husbands' active
involvement in medical care, while husbands expressed the importance
of wives being available to the family. This indicates that marital
quality is not only about whether partners support each other or not, but
also whether they are giving support that they perceive as appropriate.

Conclusion

Despite an emerging picture of the chronic illness affecting the quality of relationships, the information must be evaluated with care. The research often asks 'parents' (usually only mothers) to remember what their relationship was like before diagnosis, so it can become difficult to know how any dissatisfaction is affected by the child's illness as memory may be distorted by subsequent experiences, or if it is simply a reflection of the mother's own views. However, such research does highlight the problems that may impact on the relationship of the parents and the subsequent ability of the child and family to cope with chronic illness.

Siblings

When a child in a family is diagnosed with a chronic illness it affects the whole family. The literature tends to concentrate on the parents, but the presence of a chronically ill child has an impact on all family members including any siblings who can themselves make a significant contribution to care.

Having a chronically ill brother or sister is potentially one of the most stressful events experienced by healthy children (Drotar and Crawford, 1985). Parents invariably give their time to the sick child and even in a family receiving supportive services the needs of siblings and the impact of their contribution to the family can tend to be overlooked (Atkinson and Crawforth, 1995).

Effect on the siblings of the family

Although the parent/child relationship within a family is important, the sibling relationships may be even more significant (Miller, 1996). Brothers and sisters generally spend significantly more time with each other, and the quality of the relationships differ because of the relative amount of power each individual holds (Labatto, 1990). Sibling relationships are intense, long-lasting, complex and of an infinite variety, and add a dimension to a child's social development beyond that of the parent-child relationship. Some of the earliest lessons children learn about sharing, competition, rivalry and compromise are learnt through sibling relationships (Powell and Gallagher, 1993). Children form bonds and nurture each other, as Carr-Gregg and White (1987) concluded:

'They are obligatory relationships where, for better or worse,

> *the children spend more time together than any other family subsystem... they may assume a variety of roles with each other: mentor, supporter, comforter, protector and socialiser.'*

Siblings can provide a source of support to the family; taking on care roles and providing emotional support to the ill child, and can be a key part of a family's adaptation to the chronic illness. However, relationships between siblings are rarely static and they display varying degrees of loyalty, companionship, rivalry, love, hate, jealousy and envy (Walker, 1990). The presence of a chronic illness can affect relationships both directly and indirectly: directly, as opportunities for playing together are reduced and anxieties over illness dominate the relationship; indirectly, if the non-affected siblings feel excluded because the parents are preoccupied with the sick child, leaving little time for them. Such differential treatment can be a source of conflict, creating additional problems for the parents and for successful family adaptation. Although emphasis tends to be placed on the negative consequences for sibling behaviour, siblings can also be a source of help and support taking on aspects of care for the sick child. Thus, the sibling relationship has a potential for either positive or negative consequences for family relationships and family adaptation to chronic illness.

Impact of chronic illness on the siblings

Early research from Britain and America has tended to assume that the effect of chronic illness on the sibling will be negative, causing psychological and behavioural problems which will affect later life. But much of the research evidence was based on mothers' reports and lacked 'normal' comparative groups (Garth, 1974), and later studies, which attempted to question the children directly, have identified positive aspects such as increased empathy and kindness towards others, and greater maturity (Miller, 1996).

The reasons why some siblings have positive traits and others demonstrate behavioural difficulties is unclear, but the wide variation in response suggests that there are factors other than the presence of the disease which affect sibling behaviour (Eiser, 1993). A number of aspects have been identified in the literature as having an impact on sibling adaptation, and these include the following:

- parental reaction, with the level of acceptance and support, particularly by the mother, being significant in the response of the siblings to the sick child

- birth order, with some evidence that adverse effects are more likely to occur in younger siblings (whose own development may be jeopardised) and siblings (particularly girls) who are older than the disabled child and who take on care responsibilities
- sex of the sibling, particularly same-sex siblings who may identify with the chronically ill brother or sister
- spacing in the family and family size, with siblings in larger families coping better, perhaps due to the other siblings 'spreading the burden of care' and offering each other support
- socio-economic status of the family and family size have been found to affect development of the children, with larger families and lower socio-economic status likely to increase deviancy due to the stress of limited resources
- nature of the disability, with greater likelihood of disturbances in siblings when there is a greater degree of disability.

Each of these factors plays a part in a sibling's adaptation to the chronic illness. Although evidence suggests most siblings adjust well, the effects of living with a disabled sibling could be viewed on a continuum from adaptation to maladaptation, with the relevance and significance of the factors affecting the degree of adaptation (Miller, 1996).

Effects on siblings' development

There is considerable evidence that, following diagnosis of a chronic illness, healthy siblings have begun to show a number of disturbances in behaviour. Carpenter and Sahler (1991) reported that out of a sample of 107 siblings of children with cancer, 57 per cent showed later behavioural changes. These changes included:

- emotional lability (tearful, moody, aggressive)
- negative attention-seeking behaviour
- changes in academic performance
- withdrawal
- disturbed eating patterns
- disturbed sleeping patterns
- bedwetting
- regression to earlier developmental behaviours.

All of these suggest behaviour associated with stressful events. The reasons for this behaviour in response to the stress is unclear, although

Eiser (1993) suggested that it could be due to one of the following possibilities:

- behaviour learned from the ill child
- attention-seeking behaviour
- the sibling acting out their concerns and worries.

Whatever the reason, the presence of a chronically ill child can adversely affect the relationships between siblings and interfere with the development of the healthy child. In addition, the need to care for a sick child can create a shift in family hierarchies, with the sick child being treated as younger and the unaffected child being treated as older than their chronological ages, and this can impact on family dynamics and affect the development of all the children in the family (Freeman and Hagan, 1990). If families are to adapt successfully and meet the needs of all family members effectively, they must recognise the effects of caring for the sick child and ensure that everyone, including each sibling, is supported to meet his or her developmental potential.

Summary

The presence of a chronically ill child is potentially one of the most stressful events experienced by a healthy sibling. The focus on the ill child can result in the needs of the healthy child being neglected and so may affect his or her development. The sibling can provide a positive influence on the development of the sick child and offer support to family adaptation by taking responsibility for some aspects of care. Conversely, a sibling may hinder family coping, becoming a source of conflict due to perceived preferential treatment of the ill child.

Conclusion

The diagnosis of chronic illness disrupts family life, requiring changes to the family structure, function and role responsibilities as all members learn to cope with the demands of caring for the chronically ill child. They have to learn to share the burden of care and find ways to meet the ongoing developmental needs of all family members if they are to achieve positive adaptation to chronic illness.

Implications for practice

To enable a family to adapt to the demands of caring for a chronically ill child, practitioners need to do the following.

1 Be aware that the diagnosis of a chronic illness superimposes additional demands on the 'normal' everyday demands of family life.

2 Take account, in the assessment of a child with a chronic illness, of the changes to family roles and responsibilities resulting from caring for a chronically ill child.

3 Explore and negotiate adaptive management strategies with the family to manage the care of the sick child and the developmental needs of the other family members, such as siblings.

References

Altschuler J (1997) *Working with Chronic Illness.* Macmillan, London

Anderson JM, Elfert H (1989) Managing chronic illness in the family. Women as caretakers. *J Adv Nurs* **14**: 735–43

Atkinson N, Crawforth M (1995) *All in the Family. Siblings and Disability.* NCH, Action for Sick Children, London

Barbarin OA, Hughes D, Chesler MA (1985) Stress, coping and marital functioning among parents of children with cancer. *J Marriage and the Family* **47**: 473–80

Block HH, Block J, Morrison A (1981) Parental agreement-disagreement on child rearing orientations and gender personality correlates in children. *Child Dev* **52**: 965–74

Bradford R (1997) *Children, Families and Chronic Disease.* Routledge, London

Burr C (1985) Impact on the family of a chronically ill child. In: Hobbs N, Perrin J eds. *Issues in the Care of Children with Chronic Illness.* Jossey Bass, San Francisco

Carr-Gregg M, White L (1987) Siblings of paediatric cancer patients: a population at risk. *Med Paediatr Onc* **15**: 62–8

Carpenter PJ, Sahler OJZ (1991) Sibling perception and adaptation to chronic childhood cancer. Conceptual and methodological considerations. In: Johnson JH, Johnson SB eds. (1991) *Advances in Child Health Psychology.* University of Florida, Gainsville

Clawson JA (1996) A child with chronic illness and the process of family adaptation. *J Pediatr Nurs* **11**(1): 52–61

Cook J (1984) Influence of gender on the problems of parents of fatally ill children. *J Psychosoc Onc* **2**: 71–91

Donnelly JE, Donnelly WJ, Thong YH (1987) Parental perceptions and attitudes towards asthma and its treatment: a controlled study. *Soc Sci Med* **24**: 431–7

Drotar D, Crawford P (1985) Psychological adaptation of siblings of chronically ill children: research and practice implications. *Dev Behav Pediatr* **6**: 355–62

Eiser C (1993) *Growing up with a chronic disease. The impact on children and their families.* Jessica Kingsley Publishers, London

Freeman DJ, Hagan JW (1990) Effect of chronic childhood illness on families. *Soc Work Health Care* **14**: 37–53

Freeman H (1991) Julia. In: Cooper A, Harpin V eds. *This is Our Child. How Parents Experience the Medical World.* Oxford University Press, Oxford

Garth A (1974) Sibling reactions to mental handicap: A comparison of the brothers and sister of mongol children. *J Pediatr Nurs* **11**(5): 315–26

Gibson C (1988) Perspectives in parental coping with a chronically ill child. The case of cystic fibrosis. *Issues Comprehensive Pediatr Nurs* **11**: 33–41

Greenburg HS, Meadows AT (1991) Psychosocial impact of cancer survival on school age children and their parents. *J Psychosoc Onc* **9**(4): 43–56

Hare EH, Lawrence KM, Payne H *et al* (1966) Spina Bifida and family stress. *Br Med J* **2**: 756–60

Hauerstein E (1990) The experience of distress in parents of chronically ill children: potential or likely outcome. *J Clin Psychol* **19**: 356–64

Hornby G (1994) *Counselling in Child Disability. Skills for Working with Parents.* Chapman Hall, London

Kazak A, Marvin R (1984) Differences, difficulties and adaptation. Stress and social networks in families with a handicapped child. *Fam Relations* **33**: 67–77

Kazak A, Nachman GS (1991) Family research on childhood chronic illness: paediatric oncology as an example. *J Fam Psychol* **4**(4): 462–83

Keller S (1977) Does the family have a future? In: Skolnick A, Skolnick J *Family in transition.* 2nd edn. Boston Brown & Co, Boston

Knafl K, Brietmayer B, Zoeller L (1996) Family responses to chronic illness: a description of management styles. *J Pediatr Nurs* **11**(5): 315–26

Knafl K, Deatrick JA (1990) Family management style: concept analysis and development. *J Pediatr Nurs* **5**(1): 4–14

Labatto D (1990) *Brothers, Sisters and Special Needs.* Paul H Brookes, Baltimore

Lansky S, Cairns N, Hassanein R *et al* (1978) Childhood cancer. Parental discord and divorce. *Pediatr* **62**: 184–8

La Rossa R (1986) *Becoming a Parent.* CA Sage, Beverley Hills

Marshack LE, Seligman M (1993) *Counselling Persons with Physical Disabilities.* PRO-ED, Austin, Texas

Miller S (1996) Living with a disabled sibling - a review. *Paediatr Nurs* **8**(8): 21–4

Miller B, Wood B (1991) Childhood asthma in interaction with family, school and peer systems. A developmental model for primary care. *J Asthma* **28**(6): 405–14

Powell T, Gallagher PA (1993) *Brothers and Sisters: A Special Part of Exceptional Families.* Brookes Publishing, Baltimore

Sabbath BF, Leventhal JM (1984) Marital adjustment to chronic illness: a critique of the literature. *Pediatr* **73**: 762–8

Terkelson K (1980) Towards a theory of the family life cycle. In: Carter E, Goldrick M *The family life cycle. A framework for family therapy.* Gardner Press Inc, New York

Walker CL (1990) Siblings with cancer. *Oncol Nurs For* **17**(3): 355–60

Walker G (1991) *In the Midst of Winter.* Norton, London

Walker LS, Ford MB, Donald WD (1987) Cystic fibrosis and family stress: effects of age and severity of illness. *Pediatr* **79**: 239–46

Whall A (1986) The family as a unit of care in nursing. A historical review. *Public Health Nurs* **3**(4): 240–9

Whyte D (1992) A family nursing approach to the care of a child with a chronic illness. *J Adv Nurs* **17**(3): 317–27

Whyte D (1994) *Family Nursing: The Case of Cystic Fibrosis.* Avebury, Aldershot

Wright L, Leahey M (1990) Trends in nursing of families. *J Adv Nurs* **15**: 148–54

Additional quotes obtained through conversations with families. Names have been changed to protect confidentiality. Used with permission.

6

Family adaptation to chronic illness: learning to cope with chronic illness

Introduction

When the diagnosis of chronic illness is made the family has to come to terms with the implications of the news and also learn strategies that will help them to cope emotionally and practically with the demands of care (Altschuler, 1997). It is very important not to overemphasise the negative impact of chronic illness, but rather to explore the impact for each family. Although the process of adaptation varies with individual families, there are a number of models and frameworks that explore the issues of adaptation. These are helpful to health professionals when exploring ways to enable the family to adapt and cope effectively with the impact of having a chronically ill child.

Family adaptation

Defining family adaptation

Family adaptation models attempt to explain the effects of chronic illness in terms of homeostasis (Hornby, 1994). A family faced with the effects of chronic illness attempts to maintain a balance (homeostasis) by managing the effects of the illness on family life. The meanings families ascribe to what is happening to them (demands) and the resources they have for dealing with it (capabilities) are a critical factor in achieving a balance, which is understood in terms of family adjustment or family adaptation (Patterson, 1988).

Over time, families deal with cycles of crisis/adaptation. Some cycles are triggered by major stressors such as diagnosis, or normal developmental changes such as adolescence which may create a demand/capability imbalance and a crisis for the family. **Adaptation** is the successful resolution of the crisis by learning to cope with the demands. In contrast, **maladaptation** is when the demands are greater than the capabilities and resources of the family to cope with those demands.

The ways families deal with the stress of chronic illness vary, and some families find the problems strengthen rather than damage family bonds (Barbarin *et al*, 1985). The factors which determine why the strain affects some families in a way that leads to 'dysfunction' and others in a way that 'brings families together' are not understood (Jerrett, 1996). However, there are a number of themes and commonalties which suggest that there is a balance between 'risk factors' which create stress and 'resistance factors' which enable coping, and that this balance determines a family's degree of adjustment to chronic illness (Wallander *et al*, 1990). The factors that influence family adjustment and the degree of coping include:

- demands of the disease
- perceptions of the severity and impact of the disorder
- capabilities of the family (usually parents and siblings). The characteristics of the child, family and community can exacerbate or mediate the demands of caring for the chronically ill child.

Demands of the disease

Caring for a chronically ill child is extremely demanding both physically and emotionally. The family unit is the primary source of care for a chronically ill child and parents are taught to undertake most of the routine care (Jerrett, 1996). Yet knowing a diagnosis provides very limited information as the disease presents specific problems for each family. The demands of a disorder can vary according to its pattern, including:

- onset (gradual or sudden)
- progression (initial acute problem followed by stability, relapse or degenerative course)
- severity and frequency of symptoms
- degree of incapacity
- symptom visibility
- prognosis.

The demands of care can alter over time as the child moves through the growth and developmental stages towards adulthood, and the condition moves through a series of phases. Rolland (1987) describes the phases of illness as:

- **crisis**:
  - pre-diagnosis/diagnosis with symptoms
  - initial adjustment period
- **chronic**:
  - 'long haul' course which may be stable or degenerative
- **terminal**:
  - pre-terminal
  - death
  - terminal, mourning and resolution of loss.

Each stage presents unique tasks and requires different strengths and attitudes from the parents. The initial crisis requires the child and family to come to terms with pain, incapacitation and the implications of the disease and its treatment. This can be followed quickly by the chronic phase where the family learns to cope with the day-to-day demands of the illness in an attempt to maintain a semblance of normality. If the illness is potentially fatal then the family also has to live with the uncertainty of the disease progression and the child's eventual death.

The increase in occurrence and complexity of the care children receive at home has meant that parents have a responsibility to cope with increasingly complex care regimes. Parents become responsible for physical care-giving and have to become skilled in clinical assessment, clinical decision-making and co-ordinating care (Anderson and Elfert, 1989).

Families have to integrate the changing demands of the child with a chronic illness into family routines. Changes to everyday life can be considerable when family members learn specific skills such as physiotherapy, ensure the child is given the appropriate medication, manage changes to diet and make sure the child receives regular medical care. The physical burden of care can vary with the degree of disability and the age and size of the child. Not all conditions follow the same course and the child does not always progress at the same rate or through the 'normal' developmental stages, but parents have to learn to adapt to and cope with the changing demands of the disease and treatment as they seek to enable their child to reach their growth and development potential.

Constant vigilance

In addition to the everyday practical demands of the disease, there is a need to maintain a constant vigilance to protect the child. The uncertainty of illness can leave parents unsure of what they can trust. For example, evaluating whether a feeling of tiredness just signals that the child has worked too hard or is a recurrence of symptoms, or whether a toddler crying is an indication that their needs are unmet or indicates something more sinister, can provoke a state of constant anxiety (Altschuler, 1997). As the mother of Matthew, aged four years and being treated for leukaemia, stated:

> *'It's difficult to decide when to go to the doctor with him. I mean he's always got something. The hospital is great and don't mind if I take him if he's not well, but I don't like doing it all the time. I mean he's always got something... I feel sometimes I live there... .'*

All parents need to be aware constantly; to judge a child's needs and anticipate the consequences of actions. With chronic illness there are the additional problems of anticipating the significance of symptoms. Some disorders go through periods of stability followed by acute exacerbation. Judging if a child is genuinely ill or 'pretending', or the significance of relatively minor symptoms such as a runny nose or feeling sick, can create problems on a daily basis for all parents but these judgements can become more stressful for parents of chronically ill children when inaction may lead to severe exacerbation of the disorder. A child may appear to be in relatively 'good health', but it is sometimes difficult to judge if minor symptoms such as a cold or a sore throat in an asthmatic will clear up on their own or require treatment in order to prevent other respiratory problems.

Parents trying to judge the needs of their child, often based on inadequate information, are left uncertain of what they can trust and this leads to emotional stress and 'caregiver fatigue'. Although the results of studies of parents who are caring for children with apnoea monitors suggest the stress of care-giving decreases with time (Komelasky, 1990), these findings are not consistent with other studies which report significant caretaker fatigue (Anderson and Elfert, 1989; Ray and Ritchie, 1993). What is evident is that developmental and illness-related events can continue to impact on the stress of parents needing to 'be on call 24 hours a day' (Damrosch and Perry, 1989), and although the significance of one issue may reduce over time other problems can take on a greater importance, creating new practical and emotional demands.

Emotional demands

The emotional demands of chronic illness can also be daunting. As Eiser (1993) noted, 'Parents come to realise the ambitions they had for their child may never materialise.' A chronic illness can compromise a child's achievement by limiting experience and the acquisition of skills and this, together with periods of relapse, can add to the uncertainty about a child's future with which the parents have to learn to cope. Parents must come to terms with the knowledge that the chronic illness is for life, that the child may have to cope with painful procedures and treatments and that they will have to bear the responsibility of care. How the parents cope with emotional difficulties can determine a child's adjustment to the chronic illness.

Perceptions of the disease

There is no correlation between the severity of the disease and the ability of the family to cope or not. The experience of the illness needs to be understood in the context of the meaning for the child and family. As Benner and Wrubel (1989) stated, 'Illness as a human experience of loss or dysfunction has a reality of its own.' Thus, it is not the severity of the disease as perceived from the medical perspective, but how the families perceive the disease and the impact on their ongoing daily lives.

Communication in families can become compromised when the child has an inherited disease such as cystic fibrosis or haemophilia, with a tendency to apportion blame in attempting to come to terms with the diagnosis. However, even when conditions have no known inheritance pattern, there can still be a tendency to blame a partner. The following quote from a father of a 16 year old captures this theme:

> *'There's cancer on Joan's side, see, but, none on mine. There's no one on my side of the family who's ever had cancer; it's all Joan's side.'*

(Eiser, 1993)

The assault on self-image and self-esteem involves some deep emotions, leaving families feeling guilty and unable to cope with the suggestion that the parents cannot produce healthy children (Whyte, 1992).

Capabilities of the family

As Whyte (1997) argued, the presence of a chronically ill child can threaten the stability of the family as they adapt to the demands placed on them by the disease and subsequent treatment. Parents have to work hard to maintain the family integrity and to find time for relationships with each other, siblings and other family members. This can be problematic as the most demanding focus is often the sick child, leaving little time for anyone else.

The ability of the family to cope is influenced by the extent of such demands as work, family problems and siblings, and by the quality of support from partners. The ability to cope can be further compromised by social isolation. However, if resources are available support can be offered and utilised through the following:

- wider family network
- friends
- support groups (professional and self-help)
- educational systems
- the health care system
- social and political attitudes.

It is important to remember, however, that this support can be either helpful or obstructive. It is positive support which can enhance the family's ability to cope with the physical and emotional demands of care.

Summary

The ability of the family to adapt to chronic illness is influenced by the extent of the demands of the disease, perceptions of the disorder's severity and impact, and the capabilities of the family. Each family is unique and learns to cope with the stress of the chronic illness in a variety of ways. It is important to recognise factors that can affect family coping and adaptation to chronic illness.

Models of adaptation

There are several models which propose a theory to explain the process that people experience in their adaptation to disability, and these can provide a way to visualise how families deal with the impact of the diagnosis of chronic illness. A number of models can be found in the literature, including:

- the stage model
- the chronic sorrow model
- the developmental model.

Stage model (Hornby, 1994)

The stage model views the process of adaptation as a continuum of reactions through which people work in order to come to terms with the disability. The pattern clearly resembles a number of models of bereavement which explore the process of loss and bereavement. The stage model includes the following steps or stages experienced by individuals in the process of coming to terms with the chronic illness:

- shock
- denial
- anger
- sadness (despair or depression can also occur)
- detachment (emptiness or numbness)
- reorganisation (realism about the situation)
- adaptation (coming to terms with the situation).

As one parent commented on hearing their child's diagnosis:

> *'I have the typical reaction ... it's too bad you have to use normal words like shock, devastation, anger; but those are the words you have to use.'*

(Jerrett, 1996)

The working through of these emotions is considered to be a normal, healthy reaction to any loss; but unhealthy if the parent does not eventually come to terms with the situation. Parents may need to work through these issues several times in order to come to terms with the realisation that the child will have the illness for life. This requires that families work through and re-explore the stages of grief and loss, and has led some writers to suggest that, rather than a grieving process that can be worked through, feelings are never resolved and parents are in a constant state of sorrow (**chronic sorrow**). This becomes a part of the parents' emotional life (Thomas, 1987).

Chronic sorrow model (Fraley, 1990)

Parents feel helplessness, depression and frustration. As one parent with a child with cerebral palsy commented, 'I live with constant grief and realise now I always will to some extent' (Fraley, 1990).

Thus, although families can appear to have come to terms with the illness, at times of crisis they can bring up issues which have previously been seen to be resolved; emotions of loss and grieving. In this way, adaptation to chronic illness can be seen to be an ongoing process; parents have to learn to adapt as they face new challenges, particularly as the child progresses through the developmental stages from toddlerhood to adolescence, and problems for the child alter or become more evident as the child grows.

Developmental model (Mitchell, 1985)

The problems associated with the chronic illness and its treatment can limit a child's ability to achieve the developmental tasks expected at each age. The fact that a child is not achieving a particular developmental milestone that children of the same age have achieved, reinforces the notion that the child is different This can create stress for the parents who then come to realise that the aspirations they had for their child may never be realised (Eiser, 1993).

The family has to come to terms with the limitations of the condition and face different issues at each stage of the child's development to which they must adjust in order for both child and family to adapt successfully.

Summary

From these models it is possible to determine that adaptation to chronic illness:

- is an ongoing process
- entails some tasks the family has to achieve

- requires family members to develop coping strategies
- has the goal of 'effective' adaptation.

The goal of effective adaptation is to enable the family to manage the ongoing disease and treatment process, the child's growth and developmental needs and to maintain some sort of 'normal' family life. Each family is unique in its reaction to the different challenges of chronic illness and the responses can be adaptive, adapted in some areas and working towards adaptation in others, or ineffective management (Clawson,1996).

Families learning to cope with chronic illness

Each family needs to be assessed to determine their needs and to establish a strategy to help them adapt to the chronic illness. Canam (1993) provides an insight into the concept of adaptation and the related coping strategies. The adaptive tasks include:

- accepting the condition
- managing the condition daily
- meeting the normal developmental needs of the chronically ill child
- meeting the normal developmental needs of other family members
- coping with ongoing stress and crisis
- assisting other family members to manage feelings
- educating others about the chronic condition
- establishing support systems.

If families are to be enabled to cope it is necessary to assess their individual needs and help them to resolve issues that are potential sources of conflict.

Tasks of family adaptation

Accepting the condition

Initially the family reacts with shock and disbelief, and then denial. Giving meaning to the illness seems to facilitate family functioning, and families work hard to fit this meaning into their existing philosophy. Religious beliefs or comparing their situation can help families to come to terms with the illness. As one father commented when trying to understand why his family had a child with cystic fibrosis:

> '... I wondered if CF was given to bring us back, because we'd wandered... to bring us back to test our faith... This faith, and power and prayer, that's a great help to me.'

(Whyte, 1994)

During this time, families are often given as much information as possible to help them to come to terms with the condition. Yet there is a danger of overwhelming families with facts when they are still trying to deal with the emotional impact of the disease. As the mother of a child with cancer commented about how she felt on hearing the diagnosis:

> 'I wanted to know everything. To understand what had happened, but I can't remember what they said. People were kind but I felt in a fog... I remember having loads of leaflets... I seemed to hoard them. Over time I asked something and I got another piece of paper with information. I know I read them, but don't ask me what they said. It was that nurse who sat me down and said, "What do you need to understand?" that stopped me collecting and made me try to understand...'

Families need information, but careful consideration of what is important and what material to provide is needed. There is a danger of overwhelming parents with information which, rather than being helpful, can undermine their sense of confidence and control.

Managing the child's condition daily

For families to manage the child's condition, they need accurate and complete information at appropriate times. Part of the coping is in forming a positive relationship with the healthcare team, particularly as the family will need help in getting to know and understand the care and treatments required (Clawson, 1996). How parents are treated and supported affects how they cope with the problems. Mary, who had a son with cystic fibrosis, spoke of the strength she gained from the doctors and nurses in the hospital:

> '... *although you know they are not personal friends, you've been going there for so long and you know everyone's rooting for you.*'

(Whyte, 1994)

Meeting the child's developmental needs

This requires the family to learn how to enable the child to achieve his or her developmental potential. **Normalisation** is seen as a positive coping strategy as the parents try to engage in the usual family activities, avoiding 'special' treatment of the child. Attention is focused on what the child can or is able to do and not the disease processes.

Meeting the developmental needs of other family members

As Clawson (1996) noted, 'Family functioning seems to be the key to determining the adaptability of both the child and the family faced with the child's chronic illness.'

It is not just about meeting the needs of the child but also about ensuring that all members of the family feel supported. The key aspects that appear to determine family adaptation in meeting the needs of all family members, include:

- open communication
- sharing family responsibilities
- role flexibility
- the ability to redefine personal expectations.

All families are different and how they cope will vary, but where there is a striving for mutual support this can enable effective adaptation.

Coping with ongoing stress and periodic crises

Chronic illness as a source of stress can be both ongoing and periodic and this unpredictability can itself make the family feel anxious and vulnerable. Families need to learn coping strategies that deal with everyday problems so that a stressful event does not overwhelm their resources and lead to a crisis. They therefore need ongoing support with practical care issues and the day-to-day emotional impact of caring for the child, and not just crisis intervention.

Assisting family members to manage their feelings

Families need to identify and express how they feel, and interacting with support groups and supportive people is a way to achieve this task. Families can often become immersed in the everyday struggles, but there is also a need for them to ascribe meaning and hope to the situation. As one parent commented:

> *'I think it would be helpful if someone who had actually been through it before could be available to speak to us, really as a model of what to expect in the years to come... . Every day becomes a problem, a hassle, and I think if you can see a bit of a future ahead it helps.'*

(Hornby, 1994)

Educating others about the chronic condition

The process of being able to tell others about the child and the implications of the disorder requires that family members begin to come to terms with their child's chronic illness. Being able to have open and frank discussions with the extended family, friends and others is an important part of the process of internalising and understanding the illness.

Establishing a support system

Successful adaptation seems linked to the ability of families to share the burden of care with each other and significant others outside the family which, in turn, can minimise social isolation. As one parent stated:

> *'The most helpful support we have has come from our family*

members. If our immediate family had opted out of the situation, I think we would have been in a worse situation than it actually turned out ... .'

(Hornby, 1994)

Professionals can support the family and enable successful adaptation, but it is important to offer appropriate support. This may require an anticipation of needs in addition to addressing those issues the parents want to deal with. The perception that parents are supported, even if the services are not utilised, can be very important as the parent of a child with Down's syndrome noted:

'Professionals — well there was a lack of support in the sense that any professional contact we had, had to be initiated by us.'

(Hornby, 1994)

This family had both positive and negative experiences of professional help. However, they noted that they felt helped and supported when they had a point of contact with someone who knew what they had been through. The factors they identified as most helpful in coming to terms with the chronic illness included:

- professionals who treated them with respect and who considered the family as a whole, not just the disease
- realistic advice about what to expect and how to cope with practical problems
- being put in touch with others who 'had been through it'
- individuals who gave a perspective of hope and a future
- the provision of relevant up-to-date information and literature.

One mother stated that:

'Probably the most important thing my paediatrician did in those important early days was to place such a heavy emphasis on Natalia as a child first and foremost rather than focusing on the fact my child belonged to a population of people who were born with an extra chromosome.'

(Swirydczuk, 1991)

Not only emotional support is required, but also practical support in meeting the day-to-day needs of the child and family. Much of the burden falls to family members who have to negotiate a complex, health care system (Whyte, 1997). Families need help and support in understanding the services available to them and how to utilise them to become more self-reliant. As the mother of a child with sickle-cell disease pleads, 'Don't keep telling me what to do. Help me find it out for myself' (Davis, 1993).

If parents are to adapt to chronic illness they need an understanding of the situation and to be able to utilise strategies and resources that are effective in managing the needs of the whole family.

Conclusion

Family coping is a balancing act which attempts to manage the ongoing care of the chronically ill child, together with the effects on and the ongoing developmental needs of the whole family, and still maintain some sort of 'normality'. There are a number of adaptive tasks the family needs to work through to achieve adaptation to the presence of a chronically ill child within the unit. Adaptation to chronic illness is a complex process and if families are to achieve successful and effective adaptation they will need support that can enable them to overcome hindrances to adaptation and strengthen positive and effective coping strategies.

Implications for practice

It is important not to overemphasise the negative impact of chronic illness on family functioning, but rather to evaluate the impact for each family individually. If families are to achieve effective adaptation it is essential that they are assessed in order to determine where they have learned to cope appropriately with the implications of the chronic disorder and to identify issues that may hinder positive adaptation. Thus, practitioners need to do the following:

1   Develop an holistic perspective which recognises that the focus should always be the needs of the family and child with a chronic disease.

2   Recognise that families may need to work through their feelings and help them to find meaning in the chronic condition. This may include providing opportunities to explore previously resolved emotional issues during times of crisis.

3   Understand the importance of not overwhelming families with information or help which may initially be inappropriate to their needs. It is important to remember that needs change and families should be reassessed to ensure they have appropriate information to meet their current needs.

4   Provide parents with a 'point of contact' to discuss issues or gain information so that they can access advice or support to meet their current needs. The aim is not to make parents dependent but, through providing information or support, to give them confidence and a sense of self-reliance as they are guided through the complex health-care system

5   Ensure the family has appropriate support and resources to cope with the emotional and practical issues of day-to-day care. This may involve putting them in touch with support groups and co-ordinating services which can provide counselling, respite care, equipment or financial support.

References

Altschuler J (1997) *Working with chronic illness.* Macmillan, London

Anderson JM, Elfert (1989) Managing chronic illness in the family. Women as caretakers. *J Adv Nurs* **14**: 735–43

Barbarin OA, Hughes D, Chesler MA (1985) Stress, coping and marital functioning among parents of children with cancer. *J Marriage and the Family* **47**: 473–80

Benner P, Wrubel J (1989) *The Primacy of Caring.* Addison-Wesley, Menlo Park, California

Canam C (1993) Common adaptive tasks facing parents of children with chronic conditions. *J Adv Nurs* **18**: 46–53

Clawson JA (1996) A child with chronic illness and the process of family adaptation. *J Pediatr Nurs* **11**(1): 52–61

Damrosch SP, Perry LA (1989) Self reported adjustment, chronic sorrow and coping of parents with Down's syndrome. *Nurs Res* **38**: 25–9

Davis H (1993) *Counselling Parents of Children with Chronic Illness or Disability.* British Psychological Society, Plymouth

Eiser C (1993) *Growing Up with a Chronic Disease. The Impact on Children and Their Families.* Jessica Kingsley Publishers, London

Fraley AM (1990) Chronic sorrow: a parental response. *J Pediatr Nurs* **5**(4): 268–73

Hornby G (1994) *Counselling in Child Disability. Skills for Working with Parents.* Chapman and Hall, London

Jerrett MD (1996) Parents' experience of coming to know the care of a chronically ill child. In: Smith JP ed. *Nursing Care of Children. Advanced Nursing Series.* Blackwell Scientific Publications, London

Komelasky AL (1990) The effect of home visits on parental anxiety and CPR knowledge retention of parents of apnoea-monitored infants. *J Pediatr Nurs* **5**: 387–92

Mitchell DR (1985) Guidance needs and counselling of parents of persons with intellectual handicaps. In: Singh NN, Wilton KM eds. *Mental Retardation in New Zealand.* Whitcoulls, Christchurch

Patterson JM (1988) Chronic illness and the impact on families. In: Chilman S, Nunally EW, Cox FM eds. *Chronic illness and disability. Families in trouble.* Vol 2. Sage Publications, Newbury Park

Ray LD, Ritchie JA (1993) Chronically ill children coping at home: factors that influence parents' coping. *J Pediatr Nurs* **8**(4): 217–25

Rolland JS (1987) Chronic illness and the life cycle: a conceptual framework. *Fam Process* Vol 26: 203–21

Swirydczuk (1991) Julia. In: Cooper A, Harpin V eds. *This is our Child. How Parents Experience the Medical World.* Oxford University Press, Oxford

Thomas RB (1987) Family adaptation to a child with a chronic condition. In: Rose MH, Thomas RB eds. *Children with Chronic Conditions. Nursing in a Family Context.* Grune Stratton, Orlando

Wallander JL, Pitt LC, Mellins CA (1990) Risk factors for maladaptation in mothers of physically or sensory handicapped children: disability status, functional independence and psychological stress. *J Pediatr Psychol* **14**: 89–102

Whyte D (1992) A family nursing approach to the care of a child with a chronic illness. *J Adv Nurs* **17**(3): 317–27

Whyte D (1994) *Family Nursing: the Case of Cystic Fibrosis.* Avebury, Aldershot

Whyte D ed. (1997) *Explorations in Family Nursing.* Routledge, London

Additional quotes obtained through conversations with families. Names have been changed to protect confidentiality. Used with permission.

7

Partners in care: the participation of the child and family in care decisions

Introduction

The changes in medical treatment for children with chronic illness has meant that children are living longer, often with increasingly complex treatment regimens (Eiser, 1993). Thus, children and families with chronic illness face a lifetime of coping with illness and treatment as a result of the diagnosis. If management of the child is to be effective, then care must be viewed within a framework of partnership between the health professional and the family to ensure that care is appropriate to the family, the child and his or her ongoing developmental needs.

Partnership in care

Participation in care

Brownlea (1987) suggested that parental participation could be defined as:

> *'Parents getting involved or being allowed to become involved in a decision-making process or the delivery of care, or even simply to become one of a number of people consulted on their child's care.'*

The philosophy of participation and family-centred care has been promoted by nurses and healthcare professionals as a tenet of children's care (Coyne, 1995). This acceptance can be seen in the widening body of literature which describes involvement as partnership, and negotiation of care as desirable (Callery and Smith, 1991; Darbyshire, 1993; Neill, 1996). However, the literature focuses on parental involvement in acute hospital settings with little consideration of the wider influence of healthcare professionals in community settings or the participation of the child in decisions concerning their own care.

Participation and partnership in care are important for all families, but particularly for families with chronic illness as there is likely to be substantial contact between the family and health professionals. Yet partnership involves a major change in the roles and responsibilities of the parent, child and health professional (Callery and Smith, 1991). These changes do not operate in a vacuum as there is considerable difference in the balance of power between the child, parent and health professional. How this readjustment of the roles will be negotiated in a way that is mutually satisfying and beneficial to the child and family has been a matter of professional debate.

It could be argued that there are differences in role negotiation in hospital and home settings. Parents are in a much stronger position in their own home and have a greater degree of control and flexibility in the care of their child. However, health professionals can still exert a great deal of influence, and how the care is managed will be affected by the attitudes of the health professionals and the ways in which care is negotiated.

Negotiation of care

Negotiation of care is a recurring concept in nursing literature (Ferraro and Longo, 1985; Callery and Smith, 1991). The definition of 'to negotiate' given by the *Oxford English Dictionary* (OUP, 1971) is:

> *'to hold communication or conference (with another) for the purpose of arranging by mutual agreement; to discuss a matter with a view to some settlement or compromise.'*

However, Strauss (1978) recognised that there is no clear distinction between agreements with negotiation and agreements without negotiation, and that within healthcare other ways of obtaining a desired end can include persuasion, coercion, education and appeal to authority. The relatively stronger position of health professionals within healthcare settings often renders the child and parent dependent on the health professionals to utilise negotiation as a method for achieving a desired outcome, but it is not clear whether negotiation is always attempted by healthcare professionals (Callery and Smith, 1991).

Parental participation

There is an implicit acceptance in the literature that all parents are willing to participate in care. However, the extent to which parents are willing to participate in care is not taken into account (Darbyshire, 1993) and there has been some concern that parents may become 'reluctant collaborators' (Waterworth and Luker, 1990). Alcock, Mahoney (1990) and Cleary (1992) identified positive feelings among parents towards participation in their child's care and believe it is beneficial to the child. However, the extent to which parents want to be and are involved in their child's care varies considerably. Darbyshire (1993) found differences in the perception of partnership between parents and nurses in a hospitalised setting, with parents being willing to become involved in more aspects of care than the nurses realised. It has been noted that parents are most commonly seen as performers of tasks which vary from giving 'basic care' to becoming involved in more 'medical care' (Dearman, 1992), and that involvement was used as a tool to make the parent feel useful.

Feeling useful is seen in a number of studies as an important element in partnership (Darbyshire, 1993). As one parent explained (Gow, 1992):

> '... I felt like I shouldn't be there. The nurses were all sitting around the table and none of them came in to see us and I thought there must be nothing wrong with him and I shouldn't be there... they were all ignoring me and I didn't feel needed... I felt they were all angry because I'd gone out... maybe I'm overreacting ..., but I felt terrible.'

This demonstrates the insecurity of a parent, and also how the nursing role is perceived, which raises the question as to what extent parents can become partners and negotiate a satisfying role (Callery, 1988).

A study by Coyne (1995) illustrated that negotiation tended to evolve rather than being a product of a deliberate care plan. However, parents have to deal with experiences which to a large extent make them dependent on the flexibility and willingness of the nurse to allow them to give care. One such parent stated:

> 'There's not a lot of communication in terms of "you do this

and I'll do that"; I just do what doesn't get done, basically.'

(Coyne, 1995)

Thus, implicitly the nurse determines the role of the parents rather than exploring how care may be shared. There is an opportunity for negotiation of care to develop between health professionals and parents, particularly with chronically ill children. Care for these children is ongoing, as most chronic illnesses cannot be cured, and the family is expected to comply with complex and time-consuming treatments.

The extent to which parents are involved in care is influenced by the nurse's perception of parental competency to carry out procedures (Darbyshire, 1993). However, this is an issue of enabling the family to gain competence and confidence in caring for their child. The care of a chronically ill child is largely the responsibility of the parents and it is important that professionals recognise this and enable parents to be empowered to make decisions concerning the care of their child.

Treatment for children with chronic illness is long term and if parents are to be enabled to care for their children then health professionals need to provide support that empowers them to make informed decisions within a framework that acknowledges them as equal partners in care.

Children as partners in care

Introduction

'Children should not be just passive recipients of advice and treatment from healthcare professionals; they should play an active role in their own care.'

(Hopkins *et al*, 1994)

The focus of healthcare has been changing and patients are no longer considered to be passive, but more in control of and involved in their own healthcare. Riley (1996) believes that children should be regarded as customers too, and be able to participate and voice their opinions about the delivery of healthcare. This theme is echoed in a large body of literature (Charles-Edwards, 1991; Alderson, 1993; Kurtz, 1994; Fulton, 1996), with children perceived as having a right to participate in decisions concerning their own care. As The Children Act (1989) states:

> *'... children must be kept informed about what happens to them and participate when decisions are made about their future.'*

The ethos of the Act indicates that children are people with rights and they should have their feelings taken into account. Yet Pithers (1994) expresses concern that although rights are at the heart of The Children Act, this is more of an interpretation of intention than a reflection of what really happens.

In the exercise of children's rights, healthcare still has a long way to go. Early indications from this author's research into children with chronic illnesses are that children's participation is not guaranteed and it is largely at the discretion of the health professional. Thus, despite the considerable literature recommending that children should participate in their own care, the opportunity may not always be given to them. Yet Kurtz (1994) believes that children should be given the opportunities to acquire skills in the exercise of responsibility which will enable them to maintain their own health.

Improving compliance

The lives of children with chronic illness have been prolonged and improved due to advances in healthcare (Thompson and Gustafson, 1996), and careful compliance with care regimens is seen as the key to promoting the quality of these children's lives. However, the non-compliance of children with chronic illness is well recognised, particularly amongst the adolescent population. Dunbar-Jacob, Dunnin and Dwyer (1993) estimated that the non-compliance rate was at least fifty per cent in the paediatric population.

There is considerable evidence in the literature of adult patients that adherence to and understanding of treatment, and self-determination as well as professional respect, influences rehabilitation (Ley, 1988). More recent research has shown similar effects in children. Lewis and Lewis (1990) reported that children with asthma and epilepsy significantly improved their ability to manage health problems when they were directly involved in developing their own healthcare plan.

Although there is a widespread belief amongst practitioners that the assuming of greater responsibility for self-care by children would mean less mistakes and a greater degree of compliance through enhanced self-esteem and emotional adjustment, the empirical evidence is inconclusive.

The evidence suggests that the relationship of compliance and control is not straightforward. Hentinen and Kyngas (1996) identified that in diabetes it is the children's values, attitudes, motivation and responsibility combined with support provided by the families, friends and healthcare professionals that affects the degree of their compliance with treatment. There is no doubt that actively involving children in their own care is of value as they learn to take responsibility for their own treatment decisions, but it is the willingness of these children to participate and the encouragement they receive from their families and healthcare professionals to take responsibility which affects children's capacity to participate in their own care decisions. Thus, for treatment to be effective, partnership with the child and family needs to be encouraged with a view to developing the child's independence. To promote partnership, the following issues which may hinder this process need to be considered:

- the child's ability to make decisions
- the family's management styles, attitudes and resources
- professional attitudes.

The child's ability to make decisions

Within children's healthcare, the philosophy of family-centred care focuses on involving the whole family in care decisions, and as such it may be argued that children are already involved in decisions concerning their care. However, Lowes (1996) believes that the potential exists for a child's autonomy to be overlooked under the umbrella of family-centred care due to the focus on the parents in making care decisions for the child. In addition, there is concern that children may not be able to make their own decisions.

Much of the debate revolves around the variables associated with decision-making in children, particularly their mental capacity, age and the nature of their illness. Children with chronic illness have periods when they are not well enough to cope with complex decisions. They are still developing and often have limited communication skills and experience to draw on to articulate their needs. As a result they are dependent on adults to interpret their needs and to involve them in decisions concerning care.

The right of children under sixteen years of age to make their own decisions about their own medical treatment was, until fairly recently, non-existent. However, following the case of Gillick v Wisbech and Norfolk AHA (1986), the principle that children under this age could consent to treatment without parental authority if they were deemed to be of sufficient maturity and understanding to do so, was established. Whether a child is 'Gillick competent' to make a decision has to be assessed on an individual basis. There is no pre-determined age at which a child will become competent and the decisions children have to make can vary in complexity.

Children with chronic illnesses often have to endure long-term and complex treatment, and it is important that they understand what is happening and learn to take responsibility for treatment that is for life. However, judging if a child is competent to make a decision concerning their care is difficult and many professionals base their decisions on the child's ability to articulate their reasons for a decision.

Weithorn and Campbell (1982), by using hypothetical treatment dilemmas, found similar levels of competence between teenagers and young adults in making reasonable decisions about treatment. Furthermore, nine year olds did not differ from older subjects in arriving at the same decision but they appeared less competent to provide reasons for how or why they made those decisions. The question to be considered, then, is: would adults be able to give comprehensive reasons for all their decisions? The answer is: probably not. Yet, despite this inconsistency it would appear that professionals have made it a prerequisite of competency in children that they give sound reasons for their choices, thereby regulating the level of their involvement in their own treatment decisions.

Participation in care is often related to whether the information is provided in a way that the child will understand according to their developmental stage. As Alderson and Montgomery (1996) stated:

> '... children's competence is affected by the way they are informed and supported or excluded or dismissed.'

Clearly an appreciation of the communication and cognitive abilities of children at each developmental stage is required, but this is not just about chronological age as some children with chronic illness have additional learning disabilities and their cognitive abilities may not correlate to the expectations for their chronological age. Therefore, the information provided for the child must take account of the child's individual needs and ability to make decisions. However, partnership is not simply about providing information; although information is an integral part of the relationship between the child and the health professional, it is only one aspect. A further issue is how the information is provided and the attitude of the health professional towards the child, particularly as there is often a tacit expectation that the child will just accept the information and comply with the recommendations without question. In this way the child is protected by the adults who make decisions on their behalf.

This protectionist philosophy, which underpins the care of children in society, views children as fragile, incompetent, powerless and unable to care for themselves. Such a paternalistic attitude can affect both parents' and health professionals' attitudes to children's participation in their own care. Endorsing this protectionist view can result in denying the child the right to become involved in their own care. This may, in turn, result in harm as the child is afforded little or no autonomy, so fostering dependence rather than independence. Thus may have been created a vicious cycle in which healthcare professionals have reinforced the child's dependence by denying the need and opportunity for the child to take responsibility in their own healthcare decisions (Chadwick and Todd, 1992).

In the proposed Children's Code (Alderson and Mongomery, 1996) it is suggested that children should be presumed competent from the age of five years. This conceptual change in which the onus is on the professional to disprove a child's competency instead of being asked to prove it, may improve a child's participation in care, particularly as competency is such a subjective concept.

There is no predetermined age at which a child becomes competent, and the variables of each situation need to be taken into account as some decisions require a higher level of understanding than others. 'Gillick competence' is a developmental concept and this is a view that appears to have been taken by the Court in re R (1991). Children's competence needs to be assessed over a long period, rather than at one particular point in time.

In chronic illness, competency should be encouraged and developed over time. It is not in the child's best interests to encourage dependency. If children have little or no involvement in decisions regarding their own care they may have difficulty in making the transition to the adult healthcare arena, having gained little or no previous experience in participating in their own care decisions.

Family management styles, attitudes and resources

Alderson (1993) declares that a child's response to medical decisions will be affected by the family's way of discussing or secreting information, which must be set against the cultural and social background of that family. Parents' initial response to a child's chronic illness may be one of protection in which they take over the care of the child's illness on the child's behalf, whereas the focus should be on teaching the child to care for him- or herself. Thus, involvement in care requires an appreciation of the need to help parents to find ways of involving their children in care and improving the children's autonomy as they grow and develop. The process of teaching will depend on the age and abilities of each child, but there are always parts of care and treatment in which even the youngest child can participate.

Professional attitudes

The decision as to whether a child is competent to make a decision concerning his or her own care is usually taken by the healthcare professional involved in the care (Alderson, 1993). It has been suggested that this can create a problem due to the potential conflict of differing priorities between the child and the healthcare professional (Charles-Edwards, 1991). The medical approach to care does not readily allow decision-making and participation by children, and doctors may consider what is in the best interests of the child medically to be a priority, rather than what is in the best interests of the child overall. In addition, children may not be seen as able to understand the complexity of decisions concerning their own care. Bluebond-Langer *et al* (1990) demonstrated that many clinicians generally underestimated children's understanding and failed to involve them in the treatment process. Although this situation is changing and there is an attempt to include the child in decisions, the parents are generally seen as having authority in the child's care, and whether the child is involved will not only depend on medical attitudes but also on parental attitudes to the involvement of the child in care.

Paternalism does, however, have its place in healthcare as children cannot always understand the value of treatment. This is particularly pertinent in cases where children have surgery, such as cardiac repair. Although these children need to be well before surgery, surgery in the short term can be very debilitating and its importance for long-term health difficult to understand. Children do need protection and all decisions should take into account a wider perspective, but without unduly compromising the child's right of autonomy. Empowering a child to make a decision should be a goal of all care, but although empowerment as a concept is prominent in the adult literature (even if not always realised), in children's care it is conspicuous by its absence.

Conclusion

Partnership with children requires considerable communication skills on the part of healthcare professionals, as children are still developing and may themselves have limited communication skills and experience to enable them to express their wants or needs. As a result, children are dependent on adults to interpret their needs, drawing out what they are saying and not imposing what the adults think or want to hear. Generally children are not involved in decisions concerning their own care but, if there is to be a change in practice, there needs to be a radical re-think of the way children with chronic illnesses are viewed and cared for. This change will occur only if healthcare professionals see children as partners in their own care.

Implications for practice

If management of the child and family with a chronic illness is to be effective, the care offered must be negotiated in partnership with the child, family and healthcare professional. This requires a radical re-thinking of the way children and families are involved in care. At present, the potential exists for the child's autonomy to be overlooked under the umbrella of family-centered care. Thus, in addition to a family-centered approach, strategies need to be developed which are child-centered and which view the child and parents as equal partners in the decision-making process. It is not only embracing a philosophy of child-centered care that is required, but also providing the support and resources that empower the child and the family to make decisions concerning their care needs.

References

Alderson P (1993) *Children's Consent to Surgery.* Open University Press, Buckingham

Alcock D, Mahoney W (1990) Parents of long stay children. *Canadian Nurse* **86**(1): 20–3

Alderson P, Montgomery J (1996) *Healthcare choices; making decisions with children.* IPPR, London

Alderson P, Montgomery J (1996) What about me? *Health Serv J* **106**(5497): 22–4

Bluebond-Langer M, Perkel D, Goerztel T (1990) Children's knowledge of cancer and its treatment. The impact of an oncology camp exercise. *J Pediatr* **116**: 207–14

Brownlea A (1987) Participation: myths, realities and prognosis. *Soc Sci Med* **25**(6): 605–14

Callery P (1988) *A Study of Role Negotiation between Nurses and Parents.* University of Manchester, MSc thesis

Callery P, Smith L (1991) A study of role negotiation between nurses and the parents of hospitalised children. *J Adv Nurs* **16**: 772–81

Chadwick R, Todd W (1992) *Ethics in Nursing Practice – A Case Study Approach.* Macmillan Press, London

Charles-Edwards I (1991) Who decides? *Paediatr Nurs* Dec: 6–8

Cleary J (1992) *Caring for Children in Hospital. Parents and Nurses in Partnership.* Scutari Press, London

Coyne IT (1995) Partnership in care: parents' views of participation in their hospitalised child's care. *J Clin Nurs* **4**: 71–9

Darbyshire P (1993) Parents, nurses and paediatric nursing: a critical review. *J Adv Nurs* **18**: 1670–80

Dearman A (1992) Perceptions of parental participation. *Paediatr Nurs* **4**(7): 6–9

Department of Health (1991) *The Children Act.* HMSO, London

Dunbar-Jacob J, Dunnin EJ, Dwyer K (1993) Compliance research in paediatric and adolescent population. Two decades of research. In: Krasnegor NP, Epstein L, Jonson SB *et al* eds. *Development Aspects of Health Compliance Behavior.* Elbaum, Hillside N J

Eiser C (1993) *Growing Up with a Chronic Illness. The Impact on Children and their Families.* Jessica Kingsley Publishers, London

Ferraro R, Longo DC (1985) Nursing care of the family with a chronically ill hospitalised child; an alternative approach. *Image* **17**(3): 77–81

Fulton Y (1996) Children's rights and the role of the nurse. *Paediatr Nurs* **8**(10): 29–31

Gillick v West Norfolk and Wisbeach AHA (1985) *All England Report* **3**

Gow D (1992) Partnership between nurses and mothers. Paper presented at the RCN Paediatric Society Conference

Hentinen N, Kyngas H (1996) Diabetic adolescent compliance with health regimens and associated factors. *Int J Nurs Stud* **33**(3): 325–37

Hopkins *et al* (1994) Role of users of healthcare in a changing quality service. *Qual Healthcare* **3**: 202–9

Kurtz Z (1994) Children's rights and healthcare. *Children and Society* **8**(2): 114–31

Lewis M, Lewis C (1990) Consequences of empowering children to care for themselves. *Pediatrician* **17**: 63–76

Ley P (1988) *Communicating with the Patient. Improving Communication and Satisfaction and Compliance.* Croom Helm, London

Lowes L (1996) Paediatric nursing and children's autonomy. *J Clin Nurs* **5**: 367–72

Neill SJ (1996) Parent participation 1; literature review and methodology. *Br J Nurs* **5**(1): 34–9

OUP (1971) *The Oxford English Dictionary.* Oxford University Press, Oxford

Pithers D (1994) Acting fair. *Nurs Times* **90**(8): 32

Re R (a minor) (wardship: medical treatment) (1991) *All England Report* **4**: 177

Riley R (1996) Children are customers too. *Br J Community Nurs* **1**: 158–9

Strauss A (1978) *Negotiation: Varieties, Contexts, Processes and Social Order.* Jossey Bass, San Francisco

Thompson J, Gustafson K (1996) *Adaptation to Chronic Illness.* American Psychological Association, Washington

Waterworth S, Luker KA (1990) Reluctant collaborators: do patients want to be involved in decisions concerning care? *J Adv Nurs* **15**: 971–6

Weithorn L, Campbell S (1982) The competency of children and adolescents to make informed decisions. *Child Dev* **53**: 1589–98

Index

H

haemophilia 32,79, 91
handicap 21
hospitalisation 29–30, 33–36, 39–40, 79
hypnosis 61

I

identity 37, 40, 42–43
imagery 58, 61
independence 43
infancy 27, 28, 29, 30, 31

L

learning to adapt 49–50
leukaemia 90
lymphoma 18

M

maladaptation x, 19, 75, 87
management
  family style of 76
  parenting style of 73–75
marital relationship 70, 77, 79
massage 61
mental disability 22
misconceptions 36, 46, 57
models x
mothering 28

N

negotiation 25, 100, 104–105
non-compliance 44

O

over-protectiveness 32

P

pain x, 30, 49, 51, 54–55, 57, 59
  acute x, 51, 60
  assessment of 54–55, 59
  chronic x, 51–52, 54–57, 60
  chronic non-malignant 51
  control 57, 59
  defining 50
  diaries 54–55
  history 54
  management of 56–57
  ongoing time limited 51
  perception of 52
  procedural 58–59
  recurrent acute 51
  relief 56, 58
painful procedures 59, 91
parental
  participation 103, 105
  relationship 72, 76, 77–78
  responsibility 77
  role 70, 74, 76–79

parenting 30, 65, 74–75
  styles 23, 41, 73–75
participation 22, 103–105, 108–111
partner relationship 78
partnership 103–106, 112
  and negotiation xi
paternalism 110, 111
peer 38–39, 44
  pressure 41
  relationships 35, 37, 44
physiological processes 42
polio 75
prejudice 24
pre-operational stage 36, 53
pre-school 34
prevalence ix ,xi, 3, 5–6, 12–14, 26
professional attitudes 111

Q

quality of life ix, 50, 56

R

regression 33
relaxation 57–58, 60
role expectations 73

S

school phobia 38
school-age children 36–37
self-concept 22
self-control 32
self-esteem 35, 37, 39, 42–43, 79, 91
self-image 91
sexual identity 41, 43
siblings 72, 80–84, 92
sickle-cell disease 100
social
  competence 37
  development 35, 37, 39
  skills 34–35, 39, 44–45
stage model 93
stereotypes 39, 70
stigma 23
storm and stress 41
survival rate ix, 3–5

T

TENS 60
toddler 30, 31–33, 34, 94
touch 60
transitional-formal stage 53
treatment, consequences of 38

V

vigilance, constant 89